Newman's

Study Guide For The Clinical Medical Assistant

CMA, RMA

Authored by Xaiver Newman RMA, AHI

Co-Authored by Regina Johnson RMA

Edited and Co-Authored by Kellie Guy

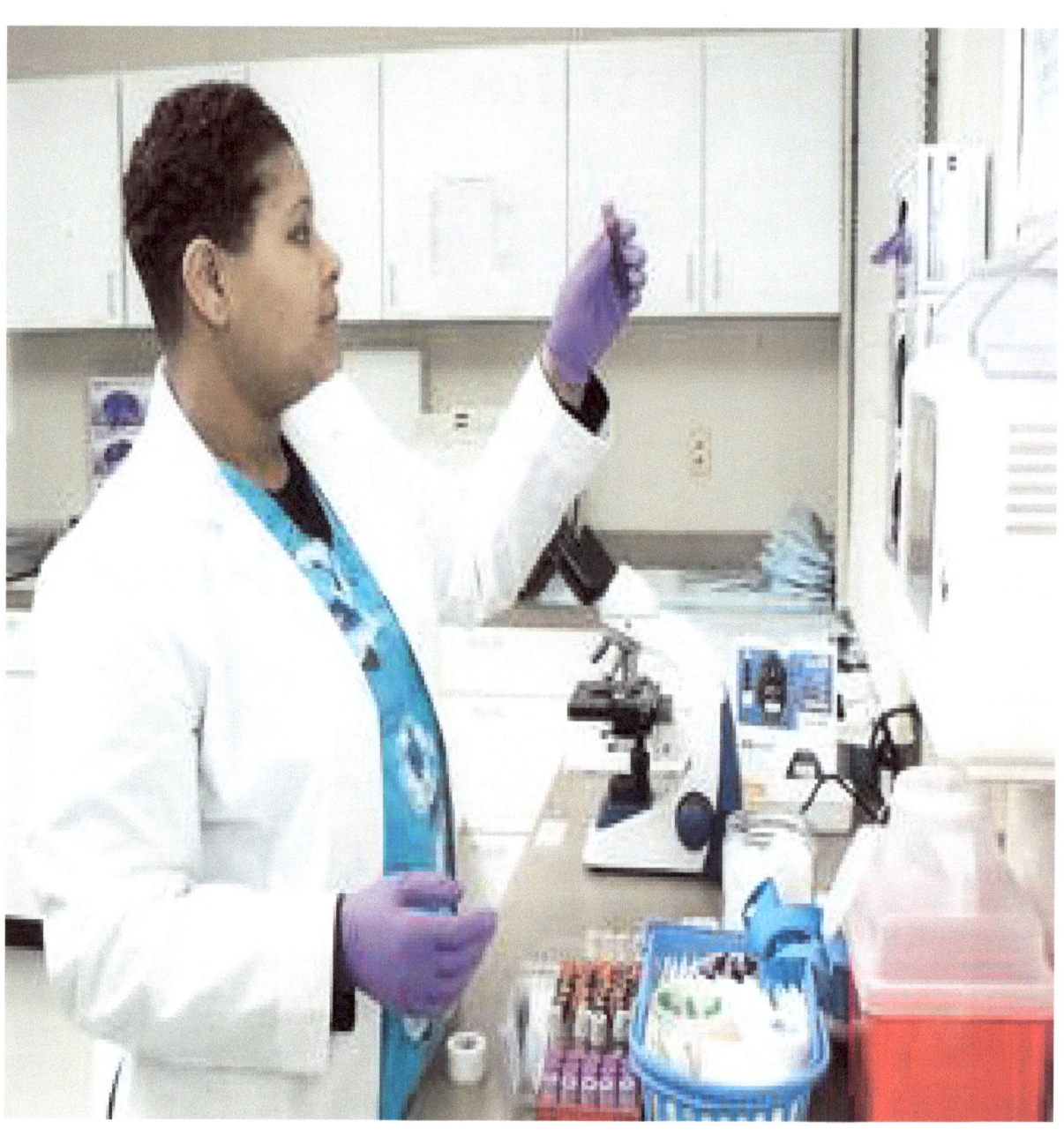

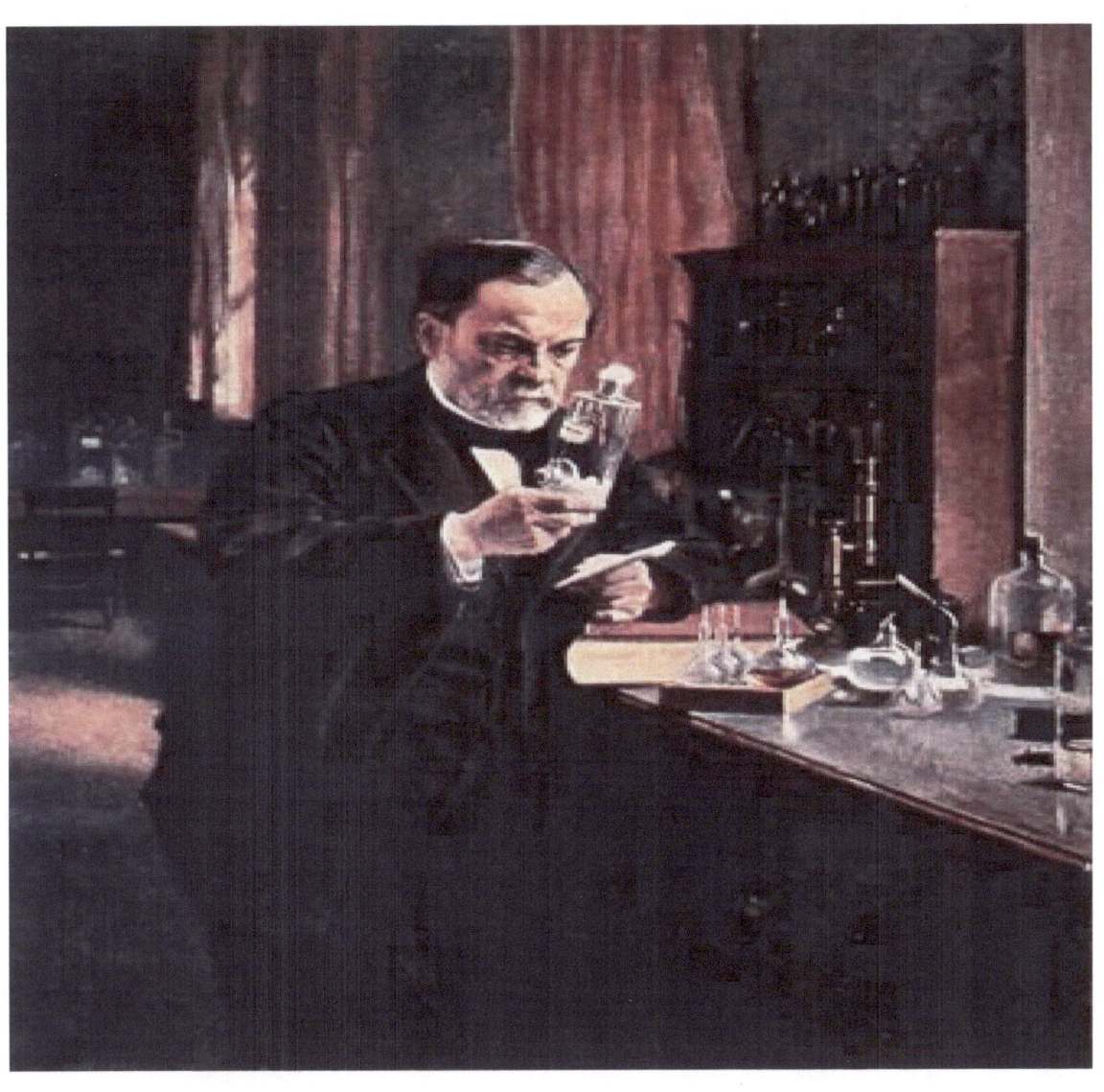

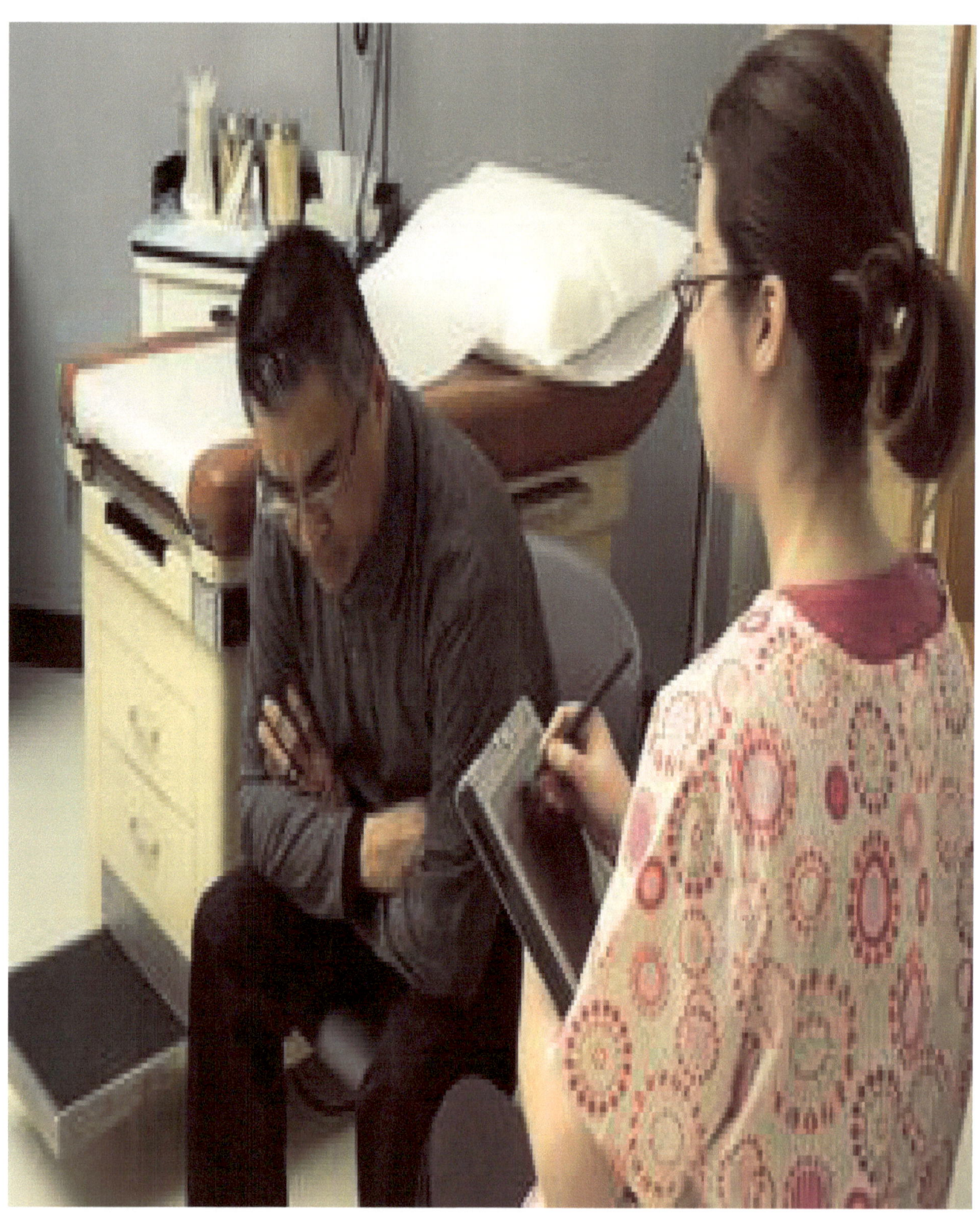

MEDICAL ASSISTANT

The Medical History	7
Vital Signs	7
Temperature	7
Pulse	8
Respiration	9
Blood Pressure	9
Common errors in blood pressure measurements:	10
Anthropometric Measurements	11
The Physical Examination	11
Positioning A Patient For Examination Or Treatment	12
Safety	14
Hazards	15
Emergency First Aid	15
Infection Control/Chain Of Infection	16
Medical Asepsis	17
Isolation Precautions	18
Latex Sensitivity	20
Parts of a Prescription	21
EKG Review	22
Anatomy of the heart	22
Figure 1: Human Heart	24
Basic Electrophysiology	25
Conduction System of the Heart	25
Figure 2: Conduction System of the Heart	26
Fundamentals of electrocardiogram	27
Figure 3: Precordial Leads	28
The electrocardiographic grid	28
Figure 4: EKG Grid	29
Waves, segments and intervals	29
The Normal Electrocardiogram Complexes	29
Artifacts	30
Stress Testing	31
Arrhythmias	31
Myocardial Ischemia and Infarction	32
Ambulatory EKG Monitoring	32
Artifacts of ambulatory EKG recording	33
Event Monitoring	33
Common Cardiovascular Agents	34
Phlebotomy Review	35
Anatomy And Physiology (An Overview)	36
The heart	36
Hemostasis	38
Site Selection	38
Venipuncture	39
Analytical Errors	44

Factors To Consider Prior To Performing The Procedure:	44
Routine Venipuncture	44
Order Of Draw	45
Failure To Obtain Blood	46
Complications Associated with Phlebotomy	46
Special Venipuncture	47
Special Specimen Handling	48
Dermal Punctures (Microcapillary collection)	48
Test Tubes, Additives And Tests	50
Clinical Laboratory Sections	52
The Microscope	54
Understanding Laboratory Measurements	54
Solutions and Dilutions	55
Arterial Blood Gas Studies	56
The Gram Stain	56
Smear Preparation	57
Urinalysis	58
General Instructions for Urine Collection	58
Types of Specimen Collection	59
Legal Considerations	62
APPENDIX A: Patients Bill Of Rights	64
References	65
Sample Test Questions	65
Answers to sample test:	69

The Medical History
Parts of the patient's medical history are:
- *Chief complaint (CC)*: the reason why the patient came to see the physician.
- *History of present illness (HPI)*: this is an explanation of the chief complaint to determine the onset of the illness; associated symptoms; what the patient has done to treat the condition, etc.
- *Past, Family and Social History* (PFSH):
  - Past medical history: includes all health problems, major illnesses, surgeries the patient has had, current medications complete with reasons for taking them, and allergies.
  - Family history: summary of health problems of siblings, parents, and other blood relatives that could alert the physician to hereditary and/or familial diseases.
  - Social history: includes marital status, occupation, educational attainment, hobbies, use of alcohol, tobacco, drugs, and lifestyles.
- *Review of Systems* - this is an orderly and systematic check of each organ and system of the body by questions. Both positive and pertinent negative findings are documented. The ROS, in conjunction with the physical examination, helps elicit information that is essential to the diagnosis of the patient's condition.

Vital Signs
Reflect the functions of three body processes necessary for life:
- Body temperature
- Respiration
- Heart function

The four vital signs of body function are:
- Temperature
- Pulse
- Respiration
- Blood pressure

Temperature
Body temperature is a balance between heat production and heat loss in conjunction with each other, maintained and regulated by the hypothalamus.

Thermometers are used to measure temperature using the Fahrenheit and Centigrade or Celsius scale. Temperature sites are the following: mouth, rectum, ear (tympanic membrane), and the axilla (underarm). The normal ranges for each site are:

Site	Normal Range
Rectal	98.6F to 100.6F (37.0C to 38.1C)
Oral	97.6F to 99.6F (36.5C to 37.5C)
Axillary	96.6F to 98.6F (35.9C to 37.0C)
Tympanic Membrane	98.6F (37C)

Some terms used to describe body temperature are:
Febrile – presence of fever
Afebrile – absence of fever

Fever – elevated body temperature beyond normal range. Types of fever are:
- Intermittent: fluctuating fever that returns to or below baseline then rises again.
- Remittent: fluctuating fever that remains elevated; it does not return to baseline temperature.
- Continuous: a fever that remains constant above the baseline; it does not fluctuate.

Oral temperature is the most common method of measurement; however, it is not taken from the following patients:
- infants and children less than six years old
- patients who has had surgery or facial, neck, nose, or mouth injury
- those receiving oxygen
- those with nasogastric tubes
- patients with convulsive seizure
- hemiplegic patients
- patients with altered mental status

Wait for 30 minutes to take the oral temperature in patients who have just finished eating, drinking, or smoking. When taking the temperature, leave the thermometer in the patient's mouth for 3-5 minutes or as required by agency policy.

Rectal temperature is taken when oral temperature is not feasible. However, it is not taken from the following patients:
- patients with heart disease
- patients with rectal disease or disorder or has had rectal surgery
- patients with diarrhea

It is taken with the patient in a side-lying position and the thermometer and the patient's hip is held throughout the procedure so the thermometer is not lost in the rectum or broken.

Axillary temperature is the least accurate and is taken only when no other temperature site can be used. The axilla, (the underarm) should be clean and dry and the thermometer should be held in place for 5-10 minutes or as required by the facility policy.

Tympanic temperature is useful for children and confused patients because of the speed of operation of the tympanic thermometer. A covered probe is gently inserted into the ear canal and temperature is measured within seconds (1–3 seconds). It is not used if the patient has an ear disorder or ear drainage.

Pulse
The normal adult pulse rate ranges between 60 and 100 beats per minute. The site most commonly used for taking pulse is the radial artery found in the wrist on the same side as the thumb. It is felt with the first two or three fingers (never with the thumb) and usually taken for 30 seconds multiplied by two to get the rate per minute. If the rate is unusually fast or slow, however, count it for 60 seconds.

The apical pulse is a more accurate measurement of the heart rate and it is taken over the apex of the heart by auscultation using the stethoscope. It is used for patients with irregular heart rate and for infants and small children.

Respiration
When measuring respiration, respiratory characteristics such as rate, rhythm, and depth are taken into account. *Rate* is the number of respirations per minute. The normal range for adults is 12 to 20 per minute. One inspiration (inhale) and one expiration (exhale) counts as one respiration. It is counted for 30 seconds multiplied by two or for a full minute.

Some rate abnormalities are the following:
   Apnea – this is a temporary complete absence of breathing which may be a result of a reduction in the stimuli to the respiratory centers of the brain.
   Tachypnea – this is a respiration rate of greater than 40/min. It is transient in the newborn and maybe caused by the hysteria in the adult.
   Bradypnea – decrease in numbers of respirations. This occurs during sleep. It may also be due to certain diseases.

Respiratory rhythm refers to the pattern of breathing. It can vary with age: infants have an irregular rhythm while adults have regular.

Some abnormalities in the rhythm are the following:
   Cheyne-Stokes – this is a regular pattern of irregular breathing rate.
   Orthopnea – this is difficulty or inability to breath unless in an upright position.

Depth of respiration refers to the amount of air that is inspired and expired during each respiration. Some abnormalities in the depth of respirations are the following:

   Hypoventilation: state in which reduced amount of air enters the lungs resulting in decreased oxygen level and increased carbon dioxide level in blood. It can be due to breathing that is too shallow, or too slow, or to diminished lung function
   Hyperpnea: abnormal increase in the depth and rate of breathing.
   Hyperventilation: state in which there is an increased amount of air entering the lungs.

Blood Pressure
This is the measurement of the amount of force exerted by the blood on the peripheral arterial walls and is expressed in millimeters (mm) of mercury (Hg). The measurement consist of two components: the highest (systole) and lowest (diastole) amount of pressure exerted during the cardiac cycle.

A stethoscope and sphygmomanometer of either aneroid or mercury type are used. The size of the cuff of the sphygmomanometer will depend on the circumference of the limb and not the age of the patient. The width of the inflatable bag within the cuff should be about 40% of this circumference – 12 cm to 14 cm in an average adult. The length of the bag should be about 80% of this circumference – almost long enough to encircle the arm. Cuffs that are too short or narrow may give falsely high readings, e.g. a regular cuff on an obese arm may lead to a false diagnosis of hypertension.

The inflatable bag is centered over the brachial artery with the lower border about 2.5cm above the antecubital crease. The cuff is positioned at heart level. If the brachial artery is far below the heart level the blood pressure will appear falsely high. If the brachial artery is far above heart level, blood pressure will appear falsely low.

Blood pressure is taken by determining first the palpatory systolic pressure over the brachial artery. Then with the bell of the stethoscope over the brachial artery, the cuff is inflated again to about 30 mm Hg above the palpatory systolic pressure and deflated slowly, allowing the pressure to drop at a rate of about 2 to 3 mmHg per second. Note the level at which you hear the sounds of at least two consecutive beats. This is the systolic pressure. Continue to lower the pressure slowly until the sounds become muffled and then disappear. Then deflate the cuff rapidly to zero. The disappearance point, which is usually only a few mmHg below the muffling point, marks the generally accepted diastolic pressure. Both the systolic and diastolic pressure levels are read the nearest 2 mmHg.

Common errors in blood pressure measurements:
- *Improper cuff size.* Cuffs that are too short or narrow may give falsely high readings. Using a regular cuff on an obese arm may lead to a false diagnosis of hypertension. For an obese arm, select a cuff with a larger than standard bag.
- *The arm is not at heart level.* If the brachial artery is much below the heart level, the blood pressure will appear falsely high. Conversely, if the artery is much above heart level, blood pressure will appear falsely low. A 13.6 cm difference between arterial and cardiac levels produces a blood pressure error of 10mmHg.
- *Cuff is not completely deflated before use.*
- *Deflation of the cuff is faster than 2-3 mmHg per second.* Rapid deflation will lead to underestimation of the systolic and overestimation of the diastolic pressure.
- *The cuff is re-inflated during the procedure* without allowing the arm to rest for 1-2 minute between readings. Repetitive inflation of the cuff can result in venous congestion, which could make the sound less audible producing artifactually low systolic and high diastolic pressure.
- *Improper cuff placement.*
- *Defective equipment.* A bag that balloons outside the cuff leads to falsely high readings.

Anthropometric Measurements

The term anthropometric refers to comparative measurements of the body. They are used as indicators of the state of health and well-being of the patient and are often included in the initial measurement of vital signs. Anthropometric measurements require precise measuring techniques to be valid.

Length, height, weight, weight-for-length, and head circumference (length is used in infants and toddlers, rather than height, because they are unable to stand) are used to assess growth and development in infants, children and adolescents. Individual measurements are usually compared to reference standards on a growth chart.

Height, weight, body mass index (BMI), waist-to-hip ratio, and percentage of body fat are the measurements used for adults. These measures are then compared to reference standards to assess weight status and the risk for various diseases.

The Physical Examination

The four principles of physical examination are:
   Inspection: which provides an enormous amount of information. The observer uses observation to detect significant physical features or objective data. This method focuses on certain aspects of the patient:
1. General appearance
2. State of nutrition
3. Body habitus
4. Symmetry
5. Posture and gait
6. Speech

Palpation: The examiner uses the sense of touch to determine the characteristics of an organ system.

Percussion - This involves tapping or striking the body, usually with the fingers or a small hammer to determine the position, size and density of the underlying organ or tissue.

Auscultation - This involves listening to sounds produced by internal organs. It is usually done to evaluate the heart, lungs, and the abdomen.

The Medical Assistant role in the physical examination:
1. Room preparation
2. Patient preparation
3. Assisting the physician

To make a diagnosis, the physician utilizes three sources: the patient's health history, the physical examination, and laboratory tests. The role of the Certified Clinical Medical Assistant during a physical examination greatly depends upon the discretion of the physician. Commonly, the Certified Clinical Medical Assistant will prepare the patient which consists of explanation and preparation, positioning, draping, vital signs, venipuncture and EKG. The Certified Clinical Medical Assistant may also prepare the room by assembling the needed instrument and equipment for the physical examination.

Positioning a Patient for Examination or Treatment
When performing an examination, treatment, tests or to obtain specimens, patients are put in special positions.

The *Horizontal Recumbent Position* is used for most physical examinations. The patient lies on his/her back with legs extended. Arms may be above the head, alongside the body or folded on the chest.

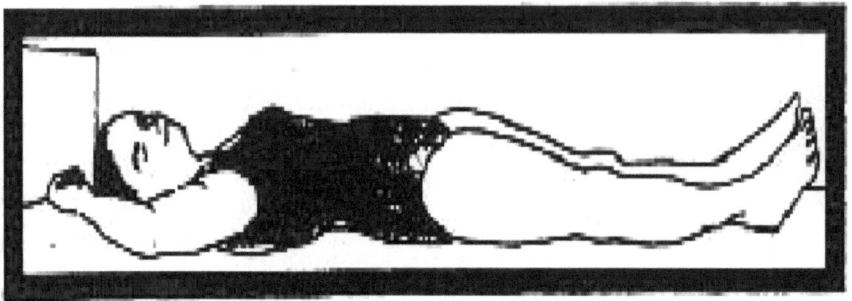

Figure 1-1. Horizontal recumbent position.

The *Dorsal Recumbent Position* is when the patient is on his/her back with knees flexed and soles of the feet flat on the bed. The MA will need to fold a sheet once across the chest and fold a second sheet crosswise over the thighs and legs so that genital area is easily exposed.

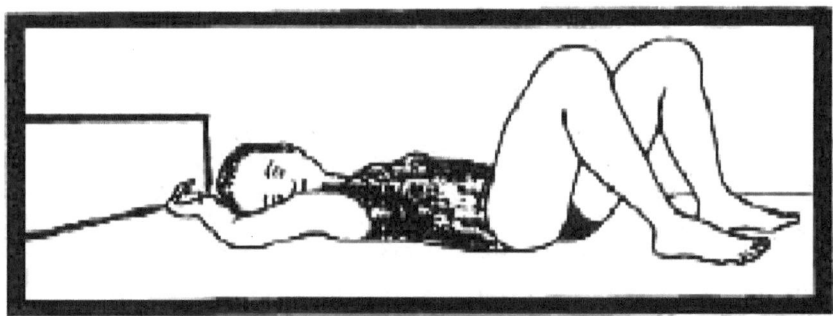

Figure 1-2. Dorsal recumbent position.

The *Fowler's Position* is used to promote drainage or to ease breathing. A sitting or semi-sitting position where the back of the examination table is elevated to either 45 degrees (Semi-Fowler's) or 90 degrees (High-Fowler's). The knees maybe raised slightly by placing a pillow underneath, but usually the legs rest flat on the table. . The patient may need a foot support. This position is usually used for patients with cardiovascular or respiratory problems, and for the examination of the upper body and head.

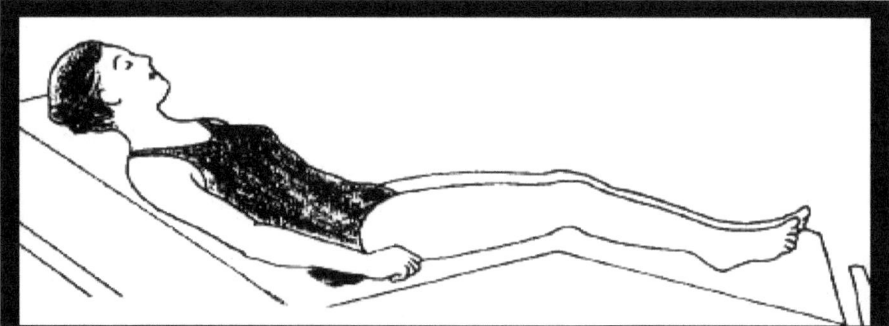

Figure 1-3. Fowler's position.

The *Dorsal Lithotomy Position* is used for examination of pelvic organs. This position is similar to the dorsal recumbent position, except that the patient's legs are well separated and thighs are acutely flexed. The feet are usually placed in stirrups and a folded sheet or bath blanket is placed crosswise over thighs and legs so that genital area is easily exposed. Keep the patient covered as much as possible.

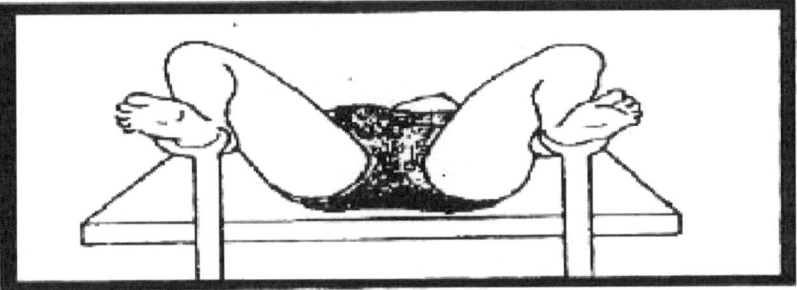

Figure 1-4. Dorsal Lithotomy position.

The *Prone Position* is used to examine the spine and back. The patient lies on his/her abdomen with head turned to one side for comfort, the arms may be above head or alongside the body. Cover with sheet or bath blanket. This position is used in the examination of the posterior aspect of the body, including the back or spine. NOTE: An unconscious patient or one with an abdominal incision or breathing difficulty usually cannot lie in this position.

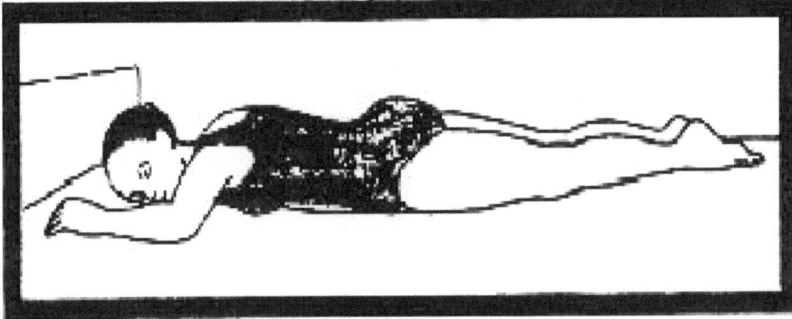

Figure 1-5. Prone position.

The *Sim's Position* is used for rectal examination. The patient is on his/her left side with the right knee flexed against the abdomen and the left knee slightly flexed. The left arm is behind the body; the right arm is placed comfortably. NOTE: Patient with leg injuries or arthritis usually cannot assume this position.

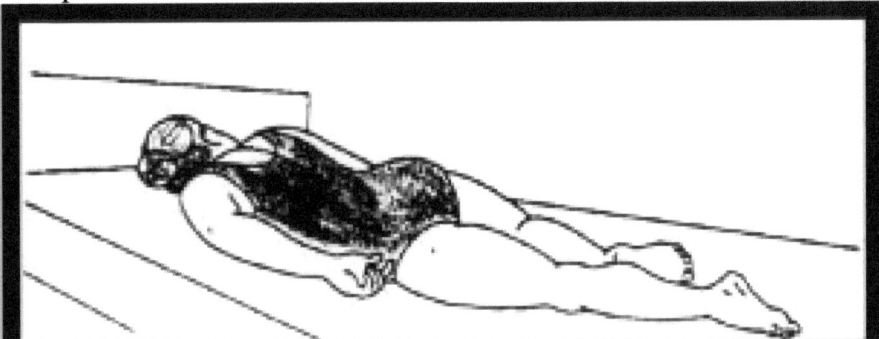

Figure 1-6. Sim's position.

The *Knee-Chest Position* is used for rectal and vaginal examinations and as treatment to bring the uterus into normal position. The patient is on his/her knees with his/her chest resting on the bed and elbows resting on the bed or arms above head. The head is turned to one side. The thighs are straight and lower legs are flat on the bed. NOTE: Do not leave patient alone; he/she may become dizzy, faint, and fall.

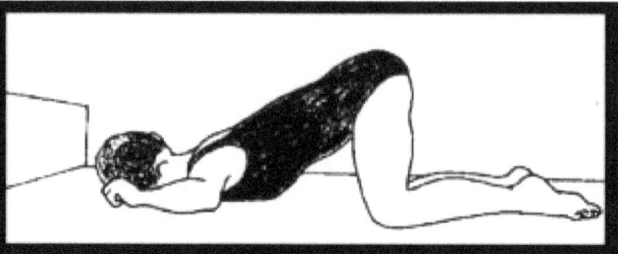

Figure 1-7. Knee-chest position.

Trendelenburg position – The patient is placed flat on the back, face up, the knees flexed and legs hanging off the end of the table, with the legs and feet supported by a footboard. The table is positioned with the head 45 degrees lower than the body. This position is used primarily for surgical procedures of pelvis and abdomen.

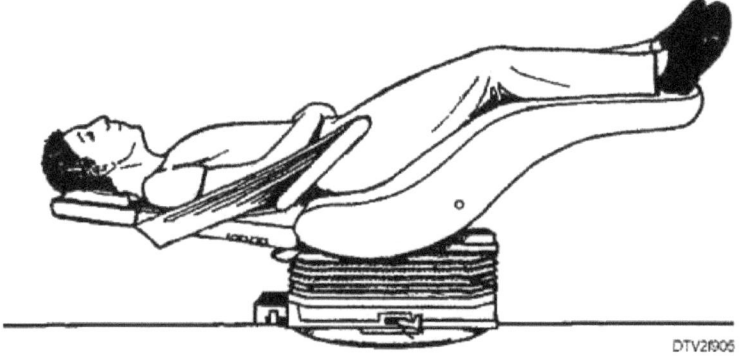

Safety

Safety hazards abound in the healthcare setting, many of which can cause serious injury or disease. The Occupational Safety and Health Administration (OSHA) is responsible for the identification of the various hazards present in the workplace and for the creation of rules and regulations to minimize exposure to such hazards. Employers are mandated to institute measures that will assure safe working conditions and health workers have the obligation to know and follow those measures.

Safety rules are usually based on common sense. Most accidents occur when these rules are neglected, overlooked or ignored. Accidents generally occur when safety is compromised because of haste and secondary shortcuts. These shortcuts can lead to personal injury and equipment damage. When an accident occurs, it **must** be reported to your supervisor immediately. Trying to cover up the incident can lead to serious, even disastrous results.

Hazards
A. Physical Hazards
  Electrical Safety Regulations
  1. Use only ground plugs that have been approved by Underwriters' Laboratory (UL).
  2. Never use extension cords.
  3. Avoid electrical circuit overloading.
  4. Inspect all cords and plugs periodically for damage.
  5. Use a surge protector on all sensitive electronic devices.
  6. Before servicing, UNPLUG the device from the electrical outlet.
  7. Use signs and/or labels to indicate high voltage or electrical hazards.

B. Chemical Hazards
  Chemical Safety Regulations
  1. If the skin or eyes come in contact with any chemicals, immediately wash the area with water for at least 5 minutes.
  2. Store flammable or volatile chemicals in a well-ventilated area.
  3. After use, immediately recap all bottles containing toxic substances.
  4. Label all chemicals with the required Material Safety Data Sheet (MDSD) information.

C. Biological Hazards
  Biological Safety Regulations
  1. Disinfect the laboratory work area before and after each use when dealing with biologicals.
  2. Never draw a specimen through a pipette by mouth. This technique is not permitted in the laboratory.
  3. Always wear gloves.
  4. Sterilize specimens and any other contaminated materials and/or dispose of them through incineration.
  5. Wash hands thoroughly before and after every procedure.

Emergency First Aid
The ability to recognize and react quickly to an emergency may be the difference of life or death for the patient. As patients react differently to various situations, it is important for all healthcare professionals to be prepared in an emergency.

External Hemorrhage: controlling the bleeding is most effectively accomplished by elevating the affected part above heart level and applying direct pressure to the wound. Do not attempt to elevate a broken extremity as this could cause further damage.

Shock occurs when there is 'insufficient return of blood flow to the heart, resulting in inadequate supply of oxygen to all organs and tissues of the body.' Patients experiencing trauma may go into shock and for some patients, seeing their own blood may induce shock. Common symptoms:
1. Pale, cold, clammy skin
2. Rapid, weak pulse
3. Increased, shallow breathing rate
4. Expressionless face/staring eyes.

   First Aid for Shock:
1. Maintain an open airway for the victim
2. Call for assistance
3. Keep the victim lying down with the head lower than the rest of the body
4. Attempt to control bleeding or cause of shock (if known)
5. Keep the victim warm until help arrives

Cardiopulmonary Resuscitation. Most healthcare institutions require their professionals to be certified in CPR. It is important for all professionals to maintain all certifications acquired.

Infection Control/Chain of Infection
This consists of links, each of which is necessary for the infectious disease to spread. Infection control is based on the fact that the transmission of infectious diseases will be prevented or stopped when any level in the chain is broken or interrupted.

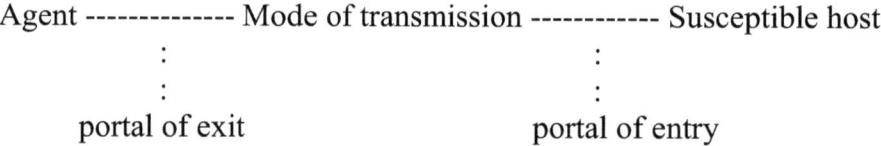

   Agents– are infectious microorganisms that can be classified into groups namely: viruses, bacteria, fungi, and parasites. When infectious diseases are identified according to the specific disease-causing microorganism, the disease may be prevented with the use of anti-infective drugs or infection control practices.

   Portal of exit –the method by which an infectious agent leaves its reservoir. Standard Precautions and Transmission-Based Precautions are control measures aimed at preventing the spread of the disease as infectious agents exit the reservoir.

   Mode of transmission –specific ways in which microorganisms travel from the reservoir to the susceptible host. There are five main types of mode of transmission:
- Contact : direct and indirect
- Droplet
- Airborne
- Common vehicle
- Vectorborne

Portal of entry – allows the infectious agent access to the susceptible host. Common entry sites are broken skin, mucous membranes, and body systems exposed to the external environment such as the respiratory, gastrointestinal, and reproductive. Methods such as sterile wound care, transmission-based precautions, and aseptic technique limit the transmission of the infectious agents.

Susceptible host – The infectious agent enters a person who is not resistant or immune. Control at this level is directed towards the identification of the patients at risk, treat their underlying condition for susceptibility, or isolate them from the reservoir.

Medical Asepsis

Best defined as "the destruction of pathogenic microorganisms after they leave the body." It also involves environmental hygiene measures such as equipment cleaning and disinfection procedures. Methods of medical asepsis are Standard Precautions and Transmission-Based Precautions.

Disinfection. This procedure used in medical asepsis using various chemicals that can be used to destroy many pathogenic microorganisms. Since chemicals can irritate skin and mucous membranes, they are used only on inanimate objects.

The least expensive and most readily available disinfectant for surfaces such as countertops is a 1:10 solution of household bleach. Boiling water (temperature of 212 F) is considered a form of disinfection, but use of it in today's medical setting is limited to items that:
1. will not be used in invasive procedures;
2. will not be inserted into body orifices nor be used in a sterile procedure

Surgical Asepsis

All microbial life, pathogens and nonpathogens, are destroyed before an invasive procedure is performed. Surgical asepsis and sterile technique are often used interchangeably.

Four methods of sterilization
1. Gas sterilization: often used for wheelchairs and hospital beds. Useful in hospitals, but costly for the office.
2. Dry heat sterilization: requires higher temperature that steam sterilization but longer exposure times. Used for instruments that easily corrodes.
3. Chemical sterilization - uses the same chemical used for chemical disinfection, but the exposure time is longer.
4. Steam sterilization (autoclave) - uses steam under pressure to obtain high temperature of 250-254F with exposure times of 20-40 minutes depending on the item being sterilized.

Handwashing

Hand washing is the most important means of preventing the spread of infection. A routine hand wash procedure uses plain soap to remove soil and transient bacteria. Hand antisepsis requires the use of antimicrobial soap to remove, kill or inhibit transient microorganisms. It is important that all healthcare personnel learn proper hand washing procedures.

Barrier Protection
Protective clothing provides a barrier against infection. Used properly, it will provide protection to the person wearing it; disposed of properly it will assist in the spread of infection. Learning how to put on and remove protective clothing is vital to insure the health and wellness of the person wearing the PPE. PPE's or personal protective equipment includes:
1. Masks
2. Goggles
3. Face Shields
4. Respirator

Isolation Precautions
For many years, the CDC recommended universal precautions, which is a method of infection control that assumed that all human blood and body fluids were potentially infectious. The CDC issued a revised guidelines consisting of two tiers or levels of precautions: Standard Precautions and Transmission-Based Precautions.

Standard Precautions
This is an infection control method designed to prevent direct contact with blood and other body fluids and tissues by using barrier protection and work control practices. Under the standard precautions, all patients are presumed to be infective for blood-borne pathogens. Infection control practices to be used with all patients. These replace universal precautions and body substance isolation. They are used when there is a possibility of contact with any of the following:

1. Blood
2. All body fluids, secretions, and excretions (except sweat), regardless of whether or not they contain visible blood
3. Nonintact skin
4. Mucous membranes designed to reduce the risk of transmission of microorganisms from both
5. Recognized and unrecognized sources of infections.

The standard precautions are:
- Wear gloves when collecting and handling blood, body fluids, or tissue specimen.
- Wear face shields when there is a danger for splashing on mucous membranes.
- Dispose of all needles and sharp objects in puncture-proof containers without recapping.

Transmission- Based Precautions the second tier of precautions and are to be used when the patient is known or suspected of being infected with contagious disease. They are to be used in addition to standard precautions. All types of isolation are condensed into three categories:

Contact precautions: are designed to reduce the risk of transmission of microorganisms by direct or indirect contact. Direct-contact transmission involves skin-to-skin contact and physical transfer of microorganisms to a susceptible host from an infected or colonized person. Indirect-contact transmission involves contact with a contaminated intermediate object in the patient's environment

Airborne precautions: are designed to reduce the risk of airborne transmission of infectious agents. Microorganisms carried in this manner can be dispersed widely by air currents and may become inhaled by or deposited on a susceptible host within the same room or over a longer distance from the source patient. Special air handling and ventilation are required to prevent airborne transmission.

Droplet precautions: are designed to reduce the risk of droplet transmission of infectious agents. Droplet transmission involves contact with the conjunctivae or the mucous membranes of the nose or mouth of a susceptible person with large-particle droplets generated from the source person primarily during coughing, sneezing, or talking. Because droplets generally travel only short distances, usually three feet or less, and do not remain suspended in the air, special air handling and ventilation are not required.

Latex Sensitivity

Latex sensitivity is an emerging and important problem in the health care field. Following the development of Universal Precaution Standards (OSHA, 1980), the use of natural rubber latex gloves for infection control skyrocketed. Within the last decade, however, the incidence of latex sensitivity has grown. Every health care worker must be concerned about latex sensitivity. Individuals with a known sensitivity to latex should wear a medical alert bracelet.

Type Reaction	Symptoms/Signs	Cause	Prevention / Management
Irritant Contact Dermatitis	Scaling, drying, cracking of skin	Direct skin irritation by gloves, powder, soaps/detergents, incomplete hand drying	Obtain medical diagnosis, avoid irritant product, consider use of cotton glove liners, consider alternative gloves/products
Allergic Contact Dermatitis (Type IV delayed hypersensitivity **or** allergic contact sensitivity)	Blistering, itching, crusting (similar to poison ivy reaction)	Accelerators (e.g., thiurams, carbamates, benzothiazoles) processing chemicals (e.g., biocides, antioxidants) Consider penetration of glove barrier by chemicals	Obtain medical diagnosis, identify chemical. Consider use of glove liners such as cotton Use alternative glove material without chemical Assure glove material is suitable for intended use (proper barrier)
NRL Allergy - IgE/histamine mediated (Type I immediate hypersensitivity) -------------------- A) Localized contact urticaria which may be associated with or progress to: B) Generalized Reaction	-------------------- Hives in area of contact with NRL -------------------- Include: generalized urticaria, rhinitis, wheezing, swelling of mouth, and shortness of breath. Can progress to anaphylactic shock	NRL proteins: direct contact with or breathing NRL proteins, including glove powder containing proteins, from powdered gloves or the environment	Obtain medical diagnosis, allergy consultation, substitute non-NRL gloves for affected worker and other non-NRL products Eliminate exposure to glove powder - use of reduced protein, powder free gloves for coworkers Clean NRL-containing powder from environment Consider NRL safe environment

Parts of a Prescription

Sample Prescription

1. The patient's name and identifying information (age, address, date of birth)
2. Today's date
3. The name of the medication
4. The dosage of the medication
5. How many doses to be taken at once
6. By what route (oral, or otherwise) the medicine should be administered
7. How often the medicine should be taken and other details about how to take it, such as time of day, or with or without food
8. The number of doses to be dispensed at once (e.g., one month supply or more)
9. Number of refills
10. DEA number
11. Doctor's signature

To understand each of these entries, some translations and explanations are necessary:
1. The patient's name should be easy to read. To better identify the patient for whom the prescription is intended, the patient's date of birth and/or address is sometimes included. Many doctors and hospitals are using typed or computer-generated prescriptions that eliminate hand-written information (except for the doctor's signature);
2. Today's date or the date the prescription was written
3. Name of the medication. To avoid names that sound alike, the generic name may appear here rather than the brand name you know. Because many medications sound alike and are spelled alike, care must be taken to make this important information clear. If a generic version or a brand name is preferred by the ordering physician, the words "no substitution" or "brand name medically necessary" may appear near the medication's name...
4. The dosage might be in milligrams (mg), micrograms (mcg), grams (g) or other unit of measure.
5. The number of doses (pills, injections, and so on) to be taken at one time, denoted as "i, ii, iii or iiii" for 1,2,3 or 4; often the term "sig" will appear just in front of these (short for the Latin, *signetur*, or "let it be labeled").

6. The mode of administration:
1. **po**: from the Latin *per os,* or "by mouth" or "orally"
2. **pr:** from the Latin *per rectum,* or "by way of the rectum," by suppository
3. **sl**: sublingual (under the tongue)
4. **IV**: intravenous
5. **IM**: intramuscular (in the muscle)
6. **SQ**: short for subcutaneous (meaning under the skin)

The frequency of administration:
1. **qd**: every day, from the Latin *quaque die,*
2. **bid**: twice a day, from the Latin *bis in die*
3. **tid**: three times a day, from the Latin *ter in die*
4. **qid:** means four times a day, from the Latin *quater in die*

If the medication is to be taken in a particular way — for example, at night or after food — that comes next:
1. **pc**: after meals or not on an empty stomach, from the Latin *post cibum*
2. **qhs:** each night, from the Latin *quaque hora somni,* or "at bedtime"
3. **prn:** as needed, from the Latin *pro re nata,* "as circumstances may require"

4. A number sign and the number of doses for the entire prescription follow. If it is a one-month supply of a medicine taken three times each day, it will read "#90"; sometimes doctors use "Disp" as shorthand for "dispense," instructing the pharmacist to provide that number of doses.
5. The number of refills allowed is next. For example, it might say "3RF" for three refills. Some prescription pads have a box for the number of doses and number of refills to be entered directly.
6. For some prescriptions, but not all, additional information is required, including doctor's Drug Enforcement Agency (DEA) number. For example, certain controlled substances, including narcotics, require a valid DEA number.
7. Finally, the doctor's name, printed and signed, complete the prescription.

EKG Review

Anatomy of the heart

The heart is a hollow muscular organ located in the thoracic cavity between the lungs just behind the sternum. The heart is actually a two-sided pump separated by a septum. The upper chambers consist of the right and left atria (singular: atrium); the lower chambers are the right and left ventricles. The chambers pump simultaneously – both atria contract together then the two ventricles

Layers of the heart
- *Endocardium* - the innermost layer of the heart. It forms the lining and folds back onto itself to form the four valves. It is in this layer that the conduction system is found.
- *Myocardium* - the middle and contractile layer of the heart. It is made up of striated muscle fibers interspersed with intercalated disks.
- *Epicardium* – the outermost layer of the heart. It is actually the inner (visceral) layer of the pericardium.

The Pericardium

The pericardium is a sac in which the heart is contained. It consists of the outermost fibrous pericardium and the serous pericardium which consists of a visceral and a parietal portion. The visceral layer invests the heart and is also called the epicardium. The parietal layer lines the fibrous pericardium. Between the visceral and parietal layers is a serous fluid which serves to prevent friction as the heart beats.

The Heart Chambers

- *Right Atrium* – receives deoxygenated blood returning to the heart from the body via the superior vena cava which carries blood from the upper body and the inferior vena cava which carries blood from the lower body.
- *Right ventricle* – receives deoxygenated blood from the right atrium which it pumps to the lungs for oxygenation through the pulmonary artery (trunk) to the right and left pulmonary arteries.
- The *pulmonary arteries* are the only arteries in the body the carry deoxygenated blood.
- *Left atrium* – receives oxygenated blood returning from the lungs via the right and left pulmonary veins.
- The *pulmonary veins* are the only veins in the body that carry oxygenated blood.
- *Left ventricle* – receives the oxygenated blood from the left atrium and pumps it to the body through the aorta, the largest artery of the body.

The Heart Valves:

The purpose of the heart valves is to prevent backflow of blood thereby assuring uni-directional flow thru the heart.

The *atrioventricular* valves (AV): so-called because they are located between the atria and ventricles.
1. Tricuspid valve – located between the right atrium and the right ventricle. As the name connotes, it has three cusps.
2. Mitral valve – located between the left atrium and the left ventricle. It has two cusps and it also called the bicuspid valve.

The *semilunar* valves: called semilunar because they have half-moon shaped cusps
- ◊ Pulmonic valve – located between the right ventricle and the pulmonary trunk.
- ◊ Aortic valve - located between the left ventricle and aorta

Murmurs are caused by diseases of the valves or other structural abnormalities. The heart sounds are produced by the closure of the valves:
- S1 – first heart sound is due to the closure of the mitral and tricuspid valves.
- S2 – second heart sound is due to the closure of the aortic and pulmonic valves.

Vessels of the Heart
The arteries supplying the heart are the right and left coronary from the aorta. The veins accompany the arteries, and terminate in the right atrium.

Neural Influences of the Heart
The heart is influenced by the autonomic nervous system (ANS) which is subdivided into the sympathetic and parasympathetic nervous systems.

Sympathetic nervous system: affects both the atria and the ventricles by increasing heart rate, conduction and irritability.

Parasympathetic nervous system: affects the atria only by decreasing heart rate, conduction and irritability.

Figure 1: Human Heart

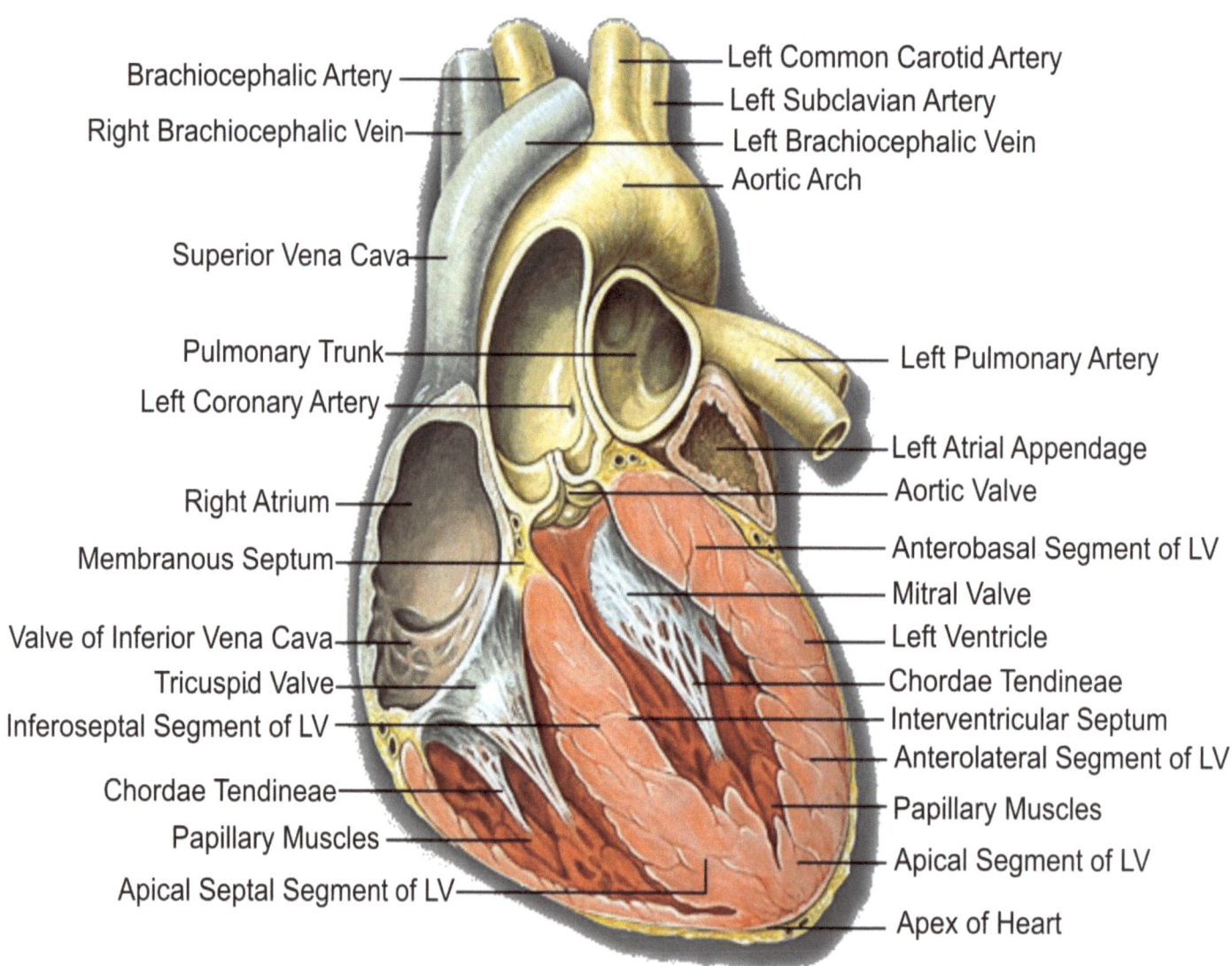

Basic Electrophysiology

Properties of cardiac cells
The primary characteristics of the cardiac cells are:
- Automaticity – This is the ability of the cardiac pacemaker cells to spontaneously initiate their own electrical impulse without being stimulated from another source. Sites that possess this characteristic are the SA node, AV junction, and the Purkinje fibers.

- Excitability – Also referred to as irritability. This characteristic is shared by all cardiac cells and it is the ability to respond to external stimulus: electrical, chemical, and mechanical.

- Conductivity – This is the ability of all cardiac cells to receive an electrical stimulus and transmit the stimulus to the other cardiac cells.

- Contractility -- This is the ability of the cardiac cells to shorten and cause cardiac muscle contraction in response to an electrical stimulus. This characteristic can be enhanced through administration of certain medications, such as digitalis, dopamine and epinephrine.

Depolarization and Repolarization
Resting cardiac cells are negatively charged inside as compared to the outside. When a cardiac cell is stimulated, sodium ions rush into the cell and potassium leaks out, changing into positive the charge within. This electrical event is called depolarization and is expected to result in contraction. Depolarization flows from the endocardium to the myocardium to the epicardium.

During cell recovery, ions shift back to their original places and the cell recovers the negative charge inside. This is repolarization, and proceeds from the epicardium towards the endocardium. It results in myocardial relaxation.

Conduction System of the Heart

SA Node
Found in the upper posterior portion of the right atrial wall just below the opening of the superior vena cava. It is the primary pacemaker of the heart and has a normal firing rate of 60-100 beats per minute.

Internodal pathways
Consists of anterior, middle and posterior divisions that distribute electrical impulse generated by the SA node throughout the right and left atria to the atrioventricular (AV) node.

AV Junction:
AV node
Located at the posterior septal wall of the right atrium just above the tricuspid valve. There is a 1/10th of a second delay of electrical activity at this level to allow blood to flow from the atria to the ventricles.

Bundle of His
Found at the superior portion of the interventricular septum, it is the pathway that leads out of the SA node. It has an ability to initiate electrical impulses with an intrinsic firing rate of 40-60 beats per minute.

Bundle branches
Located at the interventricular septum, the bundle of His divides into the right and left bundle branches, the function of which is to conduct the electrical impulse to the Purkinje fibers.

Purkinje fibers
Found within the ventricular endocardium, it consists of a network of small conduction fibers that delivers the electrical impulses to the ventricular myocardium. This network has the ability to initiate electrical impulses and act as a pacemaker if the higher level pacemakers fail. The intrinsic firing rate is 20-40 beats per minute.

Figure 2: Conduction System of the Heart

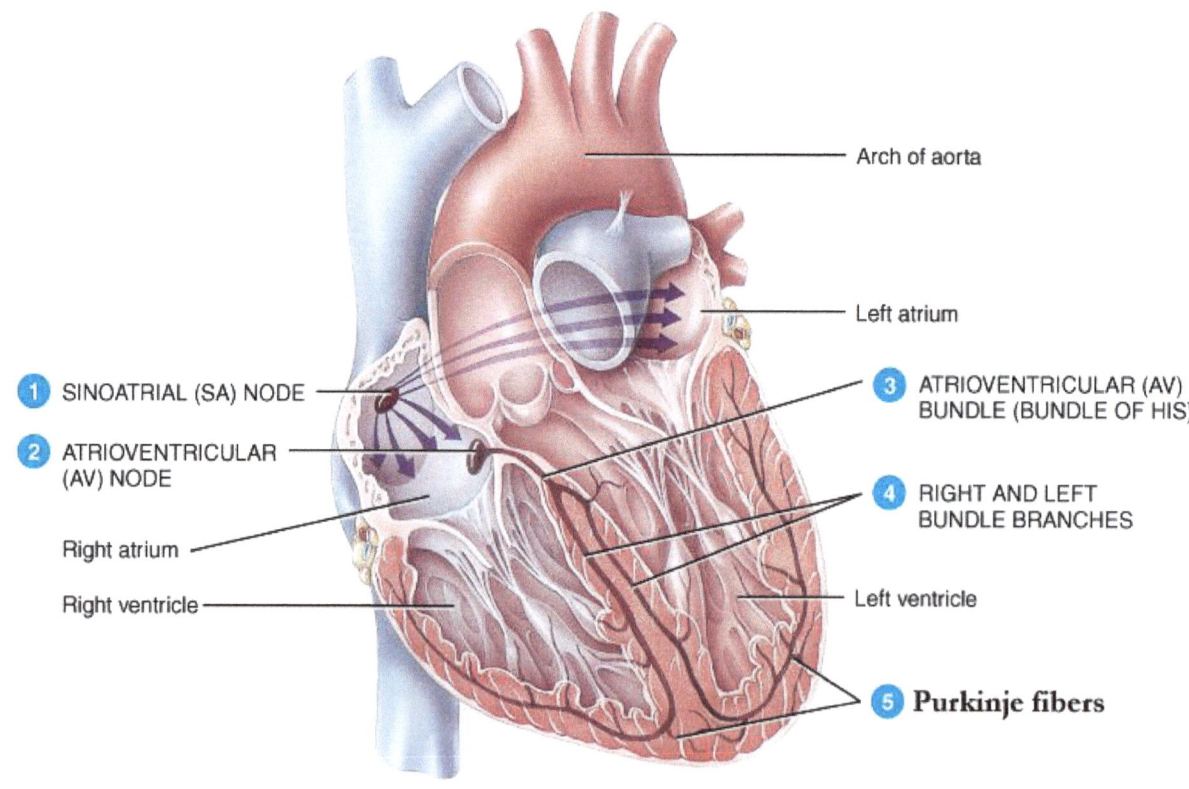

Anterior view of frontal section

Fundamentals of electrocardiogram

Limb Leads:
Consist of three bipolar leads and three augmented leads. These leads record electrical potentials in the frontal plane.

Electrodes are usually applied just above the wrists or upper arms and ankles although the electrical potential recorded will be the same no matter where electrode is placed in the extremity

Bipolar Standard Leads
Electrodes are applied to the left arm (LA), the right arm (RA) and the left leg (LL). Leads are then applied to their respective electrodes. Electrode and lead are also applied to the right leg which acts as a ground (or reference lead) and has no role in production of the electrocardiogram.

        Lead I   = the left arm is positive and the right arm is negative.
                 (LA – RA)
        Lead II = the left leg is positive and the right arm is negative.
                 (LL – RA)
        Lead III = the left leg is positive and the left arm is negative.
                 (LL – LA)

Augmented Unipolar Lead
They are designated as aVR, aVL, and aVF. These leads are unipolar and they require only one electrode from one limb to make a lead. The EKG machine uses a midpoint between the two other limbs as a negative reference point.

        Lead aVR = the right arm is positive and the other limbs are negative.
        Lead aVL =   the left arm is positive and the other limbs are negative.
        Lead aVF =   the left leg (or foot) is positive and the other limbs are negative.

Unipolar Precordial Leads
Six positive electrodes are placed on the chest to create Leads V1 through V6. They are as follows:

                      V1 : Fourth intercostal space, right sternal border.
                      V2 : Fourth intercostal space, left sternal border.
                      V3 : Equidistant between V2 and V4.
                      V4 : Fifth intercostal space, left midclavicular line
                      V5 : Fifth intercostal space, anterior axillary line
                      V6 : Fifth intercostal space, midaxillary line

Figure 3: Precordial Leads

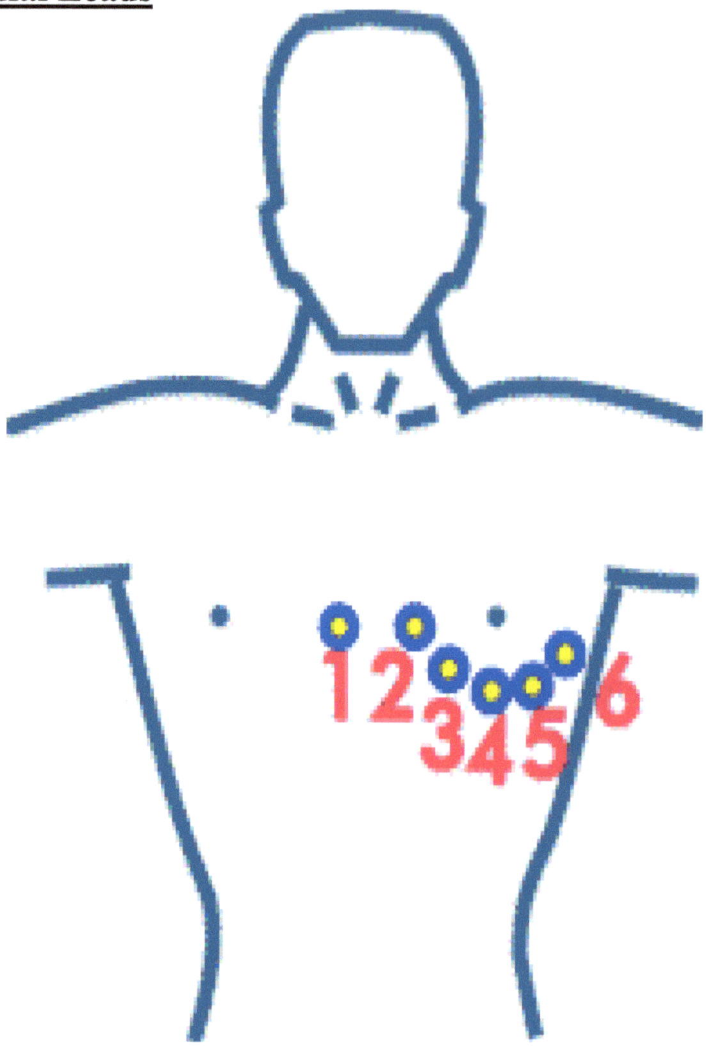

The usual routine EKG consists of placing 10 electrodes on the patient producing 12 Leads: I, II, III, aVR, aVF, aVL; V1-V6.

The electrocardiographic grid

The EKG paper is a graph paper with horizontal and vertical lines at 1-mm intervals. A heavy line appears every 5mm. The horizontal axis represents time: 1mm = 0.04 seconds; 5mm = 0.2 seconds. The vertical axis represents amplitude measured in millivolts but expressed in millimeters: 0.1mV = 1mm. The tracing is marked on the paper by a stylus using heat.

The running speed is 25mm/sec. The EKG machine must be properly standardized so that 1mV will produce a deflection of 10mm.

Figure 4: EKG Grid

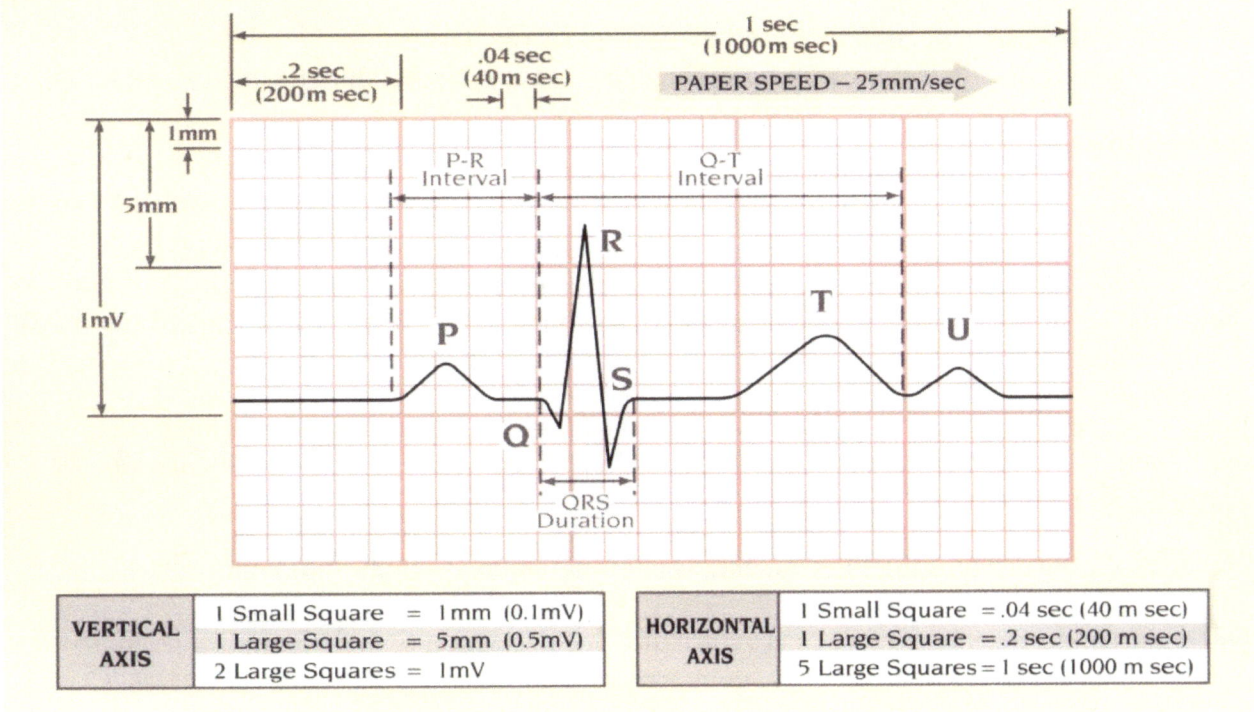

Waves, segments and intervals

1. <u>Waveform</u>: refers to movement away from the isoelectric line either upward (positive) deflection or downward (negative) deflection.
2. <u>Segment</u>: line between two waveforms.
3. <u>Interval</u>: waveform plus a segment.
4. <u>Complex</u>: several waveforms

The Normal Electrocardiogram Complexes

Atrial Activation:
1. **P wave**: the deflection produced by atrial depolarization. The normal P wave in standard, limb, and precordial leads does not exceed 0.11s in duration or 2.5mm in height.

Ventricular Activation:
2. **QRS complex**: represents ventricular depolarization (activation). The ventricle is depolarized from the endocardium to the myocardium, to the epicardium.
3. **Q (q) wave**: the initial negative deflection produced by ventricular depolarization.
4. **R (r) wave**: the first positive deflection produced by ventricular depolarization.
5. **S (s) wave**: the first negative deflection produced by the ventricular depolarization that follows the first positive deflection, (R) wave.

Ventricular Repolarization:
1. **T wave**: the deflection produced by ventricular repolarization.
2. **U wave**: the deflection seen following the T wave but preceding the next P wave.

Normal Intervals:
RR interval: this is the interval between two R waves.

If the ventricular rhythm is regular: the interval in seconds (or fraction of a second) between 2 successive R waves divided into 60 seconds = heart rate/minute. e.g. RR interval of 0.2 sec. (between two heavy lines) = 300/min heart rate; RR interval of 0.8 sec. (between 5 heavy lines) = 75/min heart rate

If the ventricular rhythm is irregular: the number of R waves in six seconds is counted and multiplied by 10 = heart rate/min e.g. 10 R waves occurred within 6 sec. = ventricular rate averages 60/min (10 x 6).

PR interval: P wave plus the PR segment. The normal interval is 0.12 – 0.2 sec.

QRS interval (or duration): represents ventricular depolarization time. It should be no more than 0.1 sec. in the limb leads and 0.11 sec. in the precordial leads.

Normal Segments and Junctions
1. PR segment: line from the end of the P wave to the onset of the QRS complex.
2. J (RST) junction: point at which QRS complex ends and ST segment begins.
3. ST segment: from J point to the onset of the T wave.

Artifacts
1. *Somatic tremors* – patient's tremors or shaking the wires can produce jittery patterns on the EKG tracing.
2. *Wandering baseline* - sweat or lotion on the patient's skin or tension on the electrode wires can interfere with the signal going to the EKG apparatus causing the baseline of the tracing to move up and down on the EKG paper.
3. *60-cycle interference* – can produce deflections occurring at a rapid rate that may mimic atrial flutter. This is caused by electrical appliances or apparatus being used nearby while the tracing is taken.
4. *Broken recording* - the stylus goes up and down trying to find the signal. This can be caused by loose electrode or cables or by frayed or broken wires.

Attention to the following will ensure against artifacts and technically poor tracings:
1. The patient should be lying on a comfortable bed or table large enough to support the entire body.
2. There must be good contact between the skin and the electrode.
3. The EKG machine must be properly standardized: 1mV should produce a deflection of 1cm (10mm).
4. The patient and the recording machine must be properly grounded to avoid alternating current interference.
5. Electronic equipment in contact with the patient can produce artifacts. i.e., IV infusion pumps

Stress Testing

A **Stress Test** is a noninvasive diagnostic procedure to determine the presence and severity of coronary artery disease. The test is performed through exercise (by having the patient walk on a treadmill or by pedaling on a bicycle), or pharmacologically (by administration of medication that causes increase in heart rate), while hooked up to an EKG monitor. The limb leads are applied to the torso of the patient rather than on the extremities themselves. A rhythm strip is run continuously throughout the test and a complete 12-lead EKG is recorded usually every 90 seconds during exercise and every minute in the recovery period post-exercise.

Some indications for stress testing are:
1. Evaluation of chest pain in patient with normal EKG.
2. Evaluation of patient who has recently had a myocardial infarction.
3. Diagnosis and treatment of arrhythmias.

Some indications for terminating the test are:
- Patient develops chest pain, shortness of breath, or dizziness.
- Blood pressure abnormalities

Exercise stress test
This test is performed until at least 85% of the target heart rate is reached or symptoms or EKG changes develop which requires the test to be terminated. Target heart rate is: 220 minus patient's age. For example, the target heart rate for a 40 year old patient is 180 (220 – 40). 85% of 180 or 153 is required for the test to be valid for interpretation.

Pharmacologic stress test
This test is appropriate for patients with physical limitation, e.g. amputees, or those who could not exercise to reach the target heart rate, e.g. elderly. Medications such as adenosine, dipyridamole, or dobutamine are given intravenously through an IV line to cause the heart rate to climb to the target level or the same symptoms and EKG changes as the exercise test develop. The test is concluded after 85% of the target heart rate is achieved.

Arrhythmias

Cardiac arrhythmias are due to the following mechanisms:
- Arrhythmias of sinus origin - where electrical flow follows the usual conduction pathway but is too fast, too slow, or irregular. Normal sinus rate is 60-100 beats per minute. If the rate goes beyond 100 per minute, it is called sinus tachycardia. If the rate goes below 60 per minute, it is referred to as sinus bradycardia.
- Ectopic rhythms - electrical impulses originate from somewhere else other than the sinus node.
- Conduction blocks - electrical impulses go down the usual pathway but encounter blocks and delays.
- Pre-excitation syndromes - the electrical impulses bypass the normal pathway and, instead, go down an accessory shortcut

Myocardial Ischemia and Infarction

Ischemia
Ischemia occurs when there is a decrease in the amount of blood flow to a section of the heart. This is usually experienced as chest pain and discomfort and is called angina.

Myocardial Infarction
Infarction refers to the actual death of the myocardial cells.

The hallmark of infarction on EKG is the presence of abnormal Q waves. Q waves are considered abnormal if they are ≥ 1 mm (0.04 second) wide and the height is greater than 25% of the height of the R wave in that lead. Q waves indicate infarcted or dead myocardial tissue. When the Q waves are combined with changes in T waves and ST segments, they indicate an acute MI.

The World Health Organization (WHO) criteria for the diagnosis of myocardial infarction are the presence of at least two of the following:
- ◊ Clinical history of ischemic-type of chest discomfort
- ◊ Changes on serial EKG tracings
- ◊ Rise and fall in serum cardiac markers

Ambulatory EKG Monitoring
Ambulatory EKG monitoring enables the evaluation of the patient's heart rate, rhythm, and QRST morphology during the usual daily activities.

Holter monitor
This is an ambulatory EKG done to rule out intermittent arrhythmias or ischemia that could be missed on a routine EKG. This may be done as an in-patient or outpatient procedure. The patient is hooked-up to a Holter monitor and EKG signals are recorded on a magnetic tape. After the prescribed duration, the patient returns the monitor to the facility and the tape is entered into a computer and scanned for abnormalities.

Five electrodes are attached to the patient's trunk instead of the arms and leg to prevent muscle artifact. The skin is prepped by abrading a thin layer of skin and then the electrodes are taped to the skin so it will adhere better and prevent from dislodging since the entire procedure will be on for 24 hours or longer. Before the ambulatory recording starts, EKG tracings are taken with the patient lying, sitting, and standing in order to be able to identify these positional changes which can bring about substantial variation in QRST morphology upon playback of the tape.

Typical electrode placement for Holter monitoring:
- Two exploring electrodes are placed over bone (to minimize motion artifact) near the V1 (over the 4th or 5th rib to the right of the sternum) and V5 (over the 5th rib at the left midaxillary line).
- Two indifferent electrodes placed over the manubrium
- One ground electrode placed over the 9th or 10th rib at the right midaxillary line

A positive Holter is one that has recorded abnormalities that may explain the patient's symptoms which could include one or more of the following:
1. Tachycardias or bradycardias
2. ST segment elevation or depression
3. Pauses

A negative Holter will have no significant arrhythmias or ST changes.

Artifacts of ambulatory EKG recording
Recording artifacts can result from the following:
- Incomplete tape erasure - this can result in EKG tracings belonging to two different patients confounding both the scanner and the interpreter.
- Tape drag within the apparatus - this will result in recording of spuriously rapid cardiac rhythms. A narrowing of all EKG complexes and intervals should give clue to this situation.
- Battery depletion - this may result in varying QRS amplitude
- Loose connection - intermittently loose connection in the insertion of the electrodes into the recording apparatus can result in the absence of all EKG signals which may mimic bradycardia-tachycardia syndrome. Clue to this artifact is the attenuated QRST morphology of the complexes beginning and ending the pause in rhythm.
- Movement of electrodes - this may occur during scratching the chest near the electrodes and can produce tracings that look like malignant ventricular arrhythmias. However, the underlying rhythm and rate remain undisturbed and should give clue to this artifact.

Event Monitoring
Some patients have symptoms very infrequently that a Holter monitor yields little useful data. These patients are best suited for an event recorder, a hand held device carried in the patient's pocket or purse which is switched only when the patient is actually experiencing the symptom. The EKG is recorded from the anterior chest wall on magnetic tape or computer chip which is scanned later the same way as that of the Holter monitor or it can be transmitted by telephone to a receiving station for immediate attention. Since the event recorder is used only when symptoms occur, multiple recording can be made over the course of a prolonged period of time.

Common Cardiovascular Agents

One of the essentials of quality care of a patient who is having an acute myocardial infarction is pharmacological therapy. The following are the common pharmacological agents used.

1. **Oxygen**

   Oxygen should be given to all patients with acute chest pain that may be due to cardiac ischemia, suspected hypoxemia of any cause, and cardiopulmonary arrest. Prompt treatment of the hypoxemia may prevent cardiac arrest. For patients breathing spontaneously, masks and nasal cannulas can be used to administer oxygen.

2. **Epinephrine**

   Epinephrine is indicated in the management of cardiac arrest. The chance of successful defibrillation is enhanced by administration of epinephrine and proper oxygenation.

3. **Isoproterenol (Isuprel)**

   Isoproterenol produces an overall increase in heart rate and myocardial contractility, but newer agents have replaced it in most clinical settings. It is contraindicated in the routine treatment of cardiac arrest.

4. **Dopamine (Intropin)**

   Dopamine is indicated for significant hypotension in the absence of hypovolemia. Significant hypotension is present when systolic blood pressure is less than 90 mmHg with evidence of poor tissue perfusion, oliguria, or changes in mental status. It should be used at the lowest dose that produces adequate perfusion of vital organs.

5. **Beta Blockers: Propranolol, Metoprolol, Atenolol, and Esmolol**

   Beta blockers reduce heart rate, blood pressure, myocardial contractility, and myocardial oxygen consumption which make them effective in the treatment of angina pectoris and hypertension. They are also useful in preventing atrial fibrillation, atrial flutter, and paroxysmal supra-ventricular tachycardia. Adverse effects of beta blockers are hypotension, congestive heart failure and broncho-spasm.

6. **Lidocaine**

   Lidocaine is the drug of choice for the suppression of ventricular ectopy, including ventricular tachycardia and ventricular flutter. Excessive doses can produce neurological changes, myocardial depression, and circulatory depression. Neurological toxicity is manifested as drowsiness, disorientation, decreased hearing ability, paresthesia, and muscle twitching, and eventual seizures.

7. **Verapamil**

   Verapamil is used in the treatment of paroxysmal supraventricular tachycardia (PSVT), effective in terminating more than 90% of episodes of PVST in adults and infants. Verapamil is also useful in slowing ventricular response to atrial flutter and fibrillation. Vigilant monitoring of blood pressure is recommended due to hypotension that could occur.

8. **Digitalis**
Digitalis increases the force of cardiac contraction as well as cardiac output. Digitalis toxicity is common with an incidence of up to 20%. Patients require constant monitoring for signs and symptoms of toxicity such as: yellow vision, nausea, vomiting, and drowsiness.

9. **Morphine Sulfate**
It is the traditional drug of choice for the pain and anxiety associated with acute myocardial infarction. In high doses, morphine sulfate may cause respiratory depression. It is a controlled substance and has a tendency for abuse and addiction.

10. **Nitroglycerin**
Nitroglycerin is a powerful smooth muscle relaxant effective in relieving angina pectoris. It is effective for both exertional and rest angina. Headache is a common consequence following the administration of this drug. Hypotension may occur and patients should be instructed to sit or lie down while taking nitroglycerin.

Phlebotomy Review

Role of the Certified Phlebotomy Technician:
1. Collect routine capillary and venous specimens for testing as requested.
2. Prepare specimen for transport, ensuring its stability.
3. Transport specimen to the laboratory.
4. Promote good public relations with hospital staff and patients.
5. Comply with new and revised procedures as described in the procedures manual.
6. Assist in collecting and documenting monthly workload and recording data.
7. Maintain safe working conditions.
8. Perform laboratory computer operations.
9. Participate in continuing education programs.
10. Perform other tasks assigned by supervisory personnel.

Professionalism
The Certified Phlebotomy Technician is a member of a service-oriented industry that requires professional behavior at all times. Professionalism is an attitude and a set of personal characteristics needed to succeed in this area. Other characteristics imperative to a Certified Phlebotomy Technician include:
- A. Dependability
- B. Honesty
- C. Integrity
- D. Empathy and compassion
- E. Professional appearance
- F. Interpersonal skills

Ethical Behavior
Ethical behavior entails conforming to a standard of right and wrong to avoid harming the patient in any way. Standards of right and wrong called the "code of ethics" provide personal and professional rules of performance and moral behavior that all Certified Phlebotomy Technicians are expected to follow.

Health Care Settings
The following are the medical facilities where the Certified Phlebotomy Technician may find work:
◊ Physician office laboratories – can range from simple screening tests done in a single practice office or specialized testing done in large group practices.
◊ Reference laboratories – These large independent laboratories perform routine and highly specialized tests that cannot be done in smaller ones. The Certified Phlebotomy Technician may do either on-site or off-site collections.
◊ Urgent care centers
◊ Nursing home facilities
◊ Wellness clinics

Anatomy and Physiology (An Overview)
This section will only touch on the basics of the anatomy and physiology of organ systems most relevant to phlebotomy, such as the heart and blood. It is highly recommended that all students who are candidates for Phlebotomy certification to have extensive knowledge of the anatomy of the heart; its' structure and function and all candidates should be prepared to demonstrate the ability to label the chambers and valves of the heart.

The circulatory system
The function of this system is to deliver oxygen, nutrients, hormones, and enzymes to the cells (exchange is done at the capillary level) and to transport cellular waste such as carbon dioxide and urea to the organs (lung and kidneys, respectively) where they can be expelled from the body. It is a transport system where the blood is the vehicle; the blood vessels, the tubes, and the heart work as the pump.

The heart
Refer to the EKG section of the study guide.

The blood vessels
The blood vessels are: Aorta, arteries, arterioles, capillaries, venules, veins, superior and inferior vena cavae.

The blood vessels, except for the capillaries, are composed of three layers. The outer connective tissue layer is called the tunica adventitia. The middle smooth muscle layer is called the tunica media. The inner endothelial layer is called the tunica intima.

The aorta, arteries, and arterioles carry oxygenated blood from the heart to the various parts of the body; while the venules, veins and the superior and inferior vena cavae carry deoxygenated blood back to the heart.

The capillaries, composed only of a layer of endothelial cells, connect the arterioles and venules. As such, capillary blood is a mixture of arterial and venous blood. The thin walls allow rapid exchange of oxygen, carbon dioxide, nutrients and waste products between the blood and tissue cells.

Blood
The average adult has 5 to 6 liters of blood. It is composed of a liquid portion called the 'plasma', and a cellular portion called the 'formed elements'. Plasma comprises 55% of the circulating blood and it contains proteins, amino acids, gases, electrolytes, sugars, hormones, minerals, vitamins, and water (92%). It also contains waste products such as urea that are destined for excretion.

The formed elements constitute the remaining 45% of the blood. They are **erythrocytes** (red blood cells), which comprise 99% of the formed elements, the **leukocytes** (white blood cells) and the **thrombocytes** (platelets). All blood cells normally originate from stem cells in the bone marrow.

The **erythrocytes** contain hemoglobin, the oxygen-carrying protein. It enters the blood as an immature reticulocyte where in one to two days, it matures into an erythrocyte. There are 4.2 to 6.2 million RBC's (red blood cells) per microliter of blood. The normal life span of an RBC is 120 days.

The **leukocytes** function is to provide the body protection against infection. The normal amount of WBC's (white blood cells) for an adult is 5,000 to 10,000 per microliter. Leukocytosis, which is an increase in WBCs, is seen in cases of infection and leukemia. Leukopenia, which is a decrease in WBCs, is seen with viral infection or chemotherapy.

There are five types of WBCs in the blood. A differential count determines the percentage of each type:

> Neutrophils – the most numerous, comprise about 40% to 60% of WBC population. They are phagocytic cells, meaning, they engulf and digest bacteria. Their number increases in bacterial infection, and often, the first one on the scene.

> Lymphocytes - the second most numerous, comprising about 20% to 40% of the WBC population. Their number increases in viral infection, and they play a role in immunity.

> Monocytes – comprising 3% to 8% of the population, they are also the largest WBCs. They are monocytes while in the circulating blood, but when they pass into the tissues, they transform into macrophages and become powerful phagocytes. Their number increases in intracellular infections and tuberculosis.

> Eosinophils - represent 1% to 3% of the WBC population. They are active against antibody-labeled foreign molecules. Their numbers are increased in allergies, skin infections, and parasitic infections.

Basophils - account for 0% to 1% of WBCs in the blood. They carry histamine, which is released in allergic reactions

The **thrombocytes** (platelets) are small irregularly shaped packets of cytoplasm formed in the bone marrow from megakaryocytes. Essential for blood coagulation, the average number of platelets is 140,000 to 440,000 per micro liter of blood. They have a life span of 9 to 12 days.

Hemostasis

Hemostasis is the process by which blood vessels are repaired after injury. This process starts from vascular contraction as an initial reaction to injury, then to clot formation, and finally removal of the clot when the repair to injury is done. It occurs in four stages:

Stage 1: Vascular phase
Injury to a blood vessel causes it to constrict slowing the flow of blood.

Stage 2: Platelet phase
Injury to the endothelial lining causes platelets to adhere to it. Additional platelets stick to the site finally forming a temporary platelet plug in a process called 'aggregation'. Vascular phase and platelet phase comprise the primary hemostasis. Bleeding time test is used to evaluate primary hemostasis.

Stage 3: Coagulation phase
This involves a cascade of interactions of coagulation factors that converts the temporary platelet plug to a stable fibrin clot. The coagulation cascade involves an intrinsic system and extrinsic system, which ultimately come together in a common pathway.

Activated partial thromboplastin time (APTT) – test used to evaluate the intrinsic pathway. This is also used to monitor heparin therapy.

Prothrombin time (PT) – test used to evaluate the extrinsic pathway. This is also used to monitor coumadin therapy.

Stage 4 – Fibrinolysis
This is the breakdown and removal of the clot. As tissue repair starts, plasmin (an enzyme) starts breaking down the fibrin in the clot. Fibrin degradation products (FDPs) measurement is used to monitor the rate of fibrinolysis.

Site Selection

The preferred site for venipuncture is the antecubital fossa of the upper extremities. The vein should be large enough to receive the shaft of the needle, and it should be visible or palpable after tourniquet placement.

Three major veins are located in the antecubital fossa, and they are:
- A. **Median cubital vein** – the vein of choice because it is large and does not tend to move when the needle is inserted.
- B. **Cephalic vein** - the second choice. It is usually more difficult to locate and has a tendency to move, however, it is often the only vein that can be palpated in the obese patient.
- C. **Basilic vein** - the third choice. It is the least firmly anchored and located near the brachial artery. If the needle is inserted too deep, this artery may be punctured.

Unsuitable veins for venipuncture are:
- A. **Sclerosed veins** - These veins feel hard or cordlike. Can be caused by disease, inflammation, chemotherapy or repeated venipunctures.
- B. **Thrombotic veins**
- C. **Tortuous veins** – These are winding or crooked veins. These veins are susceptible to infection, and since blood flow is impaired, the specimen collected may produce erroneous test results.

Note: Do not draw blood from an arm with IV fluids running into it. The fluid will alter the test results. Select another site. Do not draw blood from an artificial a-v fistula site, such as those surgically implanted in dialysis patients.

Venipuncture
The basic step in performing venipuncture is to have the necessary supplies and/or equipment organized for proper collection of specimen and to ensure the patient's safety and comfort. The recommended supplies are as follows:

- A. Laboratory requisition slip and pen.
- B. Antiseptic –
  - Prepackaged 70% isopropyl alcohol pads are the most commonly used.
  - For collections that require more stringent infection control such as blood cultures and arterial punctures Povidone-iodine solution is commonly used.
  - For patients allergic to iodine, chlorhexidine gluconate is used.
- C. Vacutainer tubes –
  - Color-coded for specific tests and available in adult and pediatric sizes.
- D. Vacutainer needles-
  - These are disposable and are used only once both for single-tube draw and multidraw (more than one tube).
  - Needle sizes differ both in length and gauge. 1-inch and 1.5-inch long are routinely used.
  - The diameter of the bore of the needle is referred to as the gauge. The smaller the gauge the bigger the diameter of the needle; the bigger the gauge the smaller the diameter of the needle (i.e. 16 gauge is large bore and 23 gauge is small bore.) Needles smaller than 23 gauge are not used for drawing blood because they can cause hemolysis.
- E. Needle adapters -

- Also called the tube holder. One end has a small opening that connects the needle, and the other end has a wide opening to hold the collection tube.
F. Winged infusion sets -
- Used for venipuncture on small veins such as those in the hand. They are also used for venipuncture in the elderly and pediatric patients.
- The most common size is 23gauge, ½ to ¾ inch long.
G. Sterile syringes and needles -
- 10-20 ml syringe is used when the Vacutainer method cannot be used.
H. Tourniquets –
- Prevents the venous outflow of blood from the arm causing the veins to bulge thereby making it easier to locate the veins.
- The most common tourniquet used is the latex strip. (Be sure to check for latex allergy). Tourniquets with Velcro and buckle closures are also available.
- Blood pressure cuffs may also be used as tourniquet. The cuff is inflated to a pressure above the diastolic but below the systolic.
I. Chux –
- An impermeable pad used to protect the patient's clothing and bedding.
J. Specimen labels -
- To be placed on each tube collected after the venipuncture.
K. Gloves -
- Must always be worn when collecting blood specimen
L. Needle disposal container –
- Must be a clearly marked puncture-resistant biohazard disposal container.
- **Never recap a needle without a safety device.**

Patient preparation procedures:

Quality control actually starts before the specimen is collected from the patient. To obtain an acceptable specimen, the patient must be prepared properly. In a hospital setting the Certified Phlebotomy Technician must check the floor book, to ensure that the nursing department has performed all pre-test preparations. Pre-test preparation will include fasting for specific tests. The Certified Phlebotomy Technician must then ensure this information is correct, by asking the patient. The Laboratory/Phlebotomy Specimen Collection Procedures Manual has established these guidelines.

Approaching a Patient
The phlebotomist uses three skills when contacting patients for phlebotomy:

- social
- clerical
- technical

Social Skills
Social skills are important. Always be polite and friendly with the patients even if they are rude or inconsiderate. Patients are often angry about their condition and take it out on the first person they see. The phlebotomist could just be waking them up or could be entering the room right after the doctor gave them bad news.

Whatever a patient says, it is inappropriate to counter with unprofessional remarks. The easiest way to defuse an upset patient is to be as polite as possible and explain that the doctor's orders need to be carried out. This social skill was outlined in the discussion of professionalism and a code of ethics in an earlier course

As the laboratory representative, the reputation of the entire laboratory rests with the phlebotomist. The patient's response to how well the laboratory performed while the patient was in the hospital is not influenced by the sophisticated instrumentation used to test the specimens. The response to friends and neighbors could be, "The blood drawers were the best I had ever seen. They were polite, skilled, and very gentle." The finest social skill guarantees this response from each patient.

Clerical Skills
Clerical skills are used constantly and contribute to the most errors in the health care setting. For the phlebotomist, the clerical skill is as simple as drawing the correct patient's blood and labeling it with the correct name. Sounds simple, but numerous errors occur in this one area.

An error can have devastating effects. The wrong patient could be drawn for a transfusion of blood. The blood would be labeled with the name of the patient you were supposed to draw but the blood in the tube would not be of that patient. The preparation of the blood for transfusion (crossmatch) would not be done on the correct blood. The patient would then receive units of blood that were not compatible. The side effects of such an error could be kidney failure or death

Here is another example of a clerical error. The right patient was drawn for blood glucose and the correct result was reported to the nursing unit. But the nurse misread the result and gave the wrong dosage of insulin.

Clerical errors can occur at any step during the care of a patient. The phlebotomist does not want to be the cause of an error. The phlebotomist's errors are usually restricted to patient misidentification or mislabeling of a blood sample.

Technical Skills
Technical skills mean obtaining blood successfully with minimal pain. They consist of whatever method is used to complete the procedure: venipuncture, arterial sample, or microcollections through skin puncture.

Social, clerical, and technical skills are used in each patient contact and are intertwined in each step of taking a blood sample. The approach to the patient often determines the success of the venipuncture. The muscles of a tense patient tighten over the blood veins, making them more difficult to access. A relaxed patient is more cooperative and easier to draw.

Patient Identification

It cannot be repeated often enough that proper patient identification is essential to accurate patient testing. It does not matter how expensive or sophisticated the equipment the sample is tested on, the results will be wrong if the sample is not identified accurately.

Most patients have a hospital identification bracelet that includes their first and last names, hospital numbers (often two sets of numbers), birthdate, and physician. When the phlebotomist enters the room, do not say "Mr. Jones, I'm here to draw your blood" and assume if the patient says "yes" he is Mr. Jones. The patient will often have been asleep or not paying attention and will answer yes even if it is Mrs. Smith in the bed

Ask the conscious patient to state his or her full name. This lets patients realize someone is in the room and it gets them thinking so they will be awake when their blood is collected. The phlebotomist still needs to check the armband to verify the correct patient is being drawn even after the patient has stated his or her name. In addition to checking the patient's name, check the patient's identification numbers.

The manual requisition is imprinted from an addressograph plate that prints the patient's name, identification numbers, physician, and room number. This plate is similar to a credit card plate, only it contains more information. The manual requisition can also be handwritten. With either method, the test required is check-marked or the required test is handwritten on the order form.

The computer label has several advantages. It lists the specific test that was ordered and the required specimen and specimen requirements. The label is usually adhesive so it can be attached directly to the tube. Smaller labels can also be printed at the same time for smaller aliquot specimens

The computer has multiple other advantages in timing the print of orders, sorting lists of orders for one patient at one time, and speeding entry of draw times and test results. Most hospitals use some type of computer system for test ordering and result reporting. The computer labels print off in a roll where one label follows the other.

The identification numbers on the patient's armband are compared to the name and numbers on the order form used in the health care institution. These order forms can be a manual requisition that is usually a multipart carbon form or an adhesive computer label as shown here:

Accessioning Order

Each request for a blood specimen must include an accessioning order: a number to identify all paperwork and supplies associated with each patient. This unique number can be used to trace back that specimen and patient. It ensures accurate and prompt processing of various forms required when performing a venipuncture and analyzing the results. The blood request forms should include the following information:

1. Patient's name and age from ID plate or wristband.
2. Identification number.
3. Date and time the specimen is obtained.
4. Name or initials of person who obtains the specimen
5. Accessioning number.
6. Physician's name.
7. Department for which work is being done.
8. Other useful information, for example, special comments: unusual sampling site, drawn near an IV site.

The blood is drawn and processed by institutional policy. Most health care areas do not label the tubes before the blood sample is drawn for outpatients. Outpatient and inpatient specimens are labeled after the specimen is drawn and before the phlebotomist leaves the patient. In each case there is a potential for a clerical error. Each tube and label must be checked to assure that proper identification is completed.

If you accession a patient in the emergency room where identification is not immediate, follow these steps:

1. Assign a master identification number (temporary) to the patient. Use a three-part identification tag with the same master number on all three parts: (a) Attach the first part to the patient's arm, (b) attach the second part to the specimen, and (c) attach the third part to the blood transfusion bag if a transfusion has been ordered.
2. Select the appropriate test forms and write the identification number on the forms.
3. Complete the necessary labels and apply to the specimens.
4. Cross-reference the permanent identification number to the temporary number after a permanent number is assigned

Analytical Errors

Before Collection:	During Collection	After Collection
Patient misidentification	Extended tourniquet time	Failure to separate serum from cell
Improper Time of Collection	Hemolysis	Improper use of serum separator
Wrong Tube	Wrong order of draw	Processing delays
Inadequate fast	Failure to invert tubes	Exposure to light
Exercise	Faulty technique	Improper storage conditions
Patient posture	Under filling tubes	Rimming clots
Poor coordination with other treatments		
Improper site preparation		
Medication interference		

Ernst, Dennis, J. Applied Phlebotomy. Lippencott Williams & Wilkins.2005

Factors to Consider Prior To Performing the Procedure:
1. **Fasting** – some tests such as those for glucose, cholesterol, and triglycerides require that the patient abstain from eating for at least 12 hours. The Certified Phlebotomy Technician must ascertain that the patient is indeed in a fasting state prior to the testing.
2. **Edema** – is the accumulation of fluid in the tissues. Collection from edematous tissue alters test results.
3. **Fistula** - is the permanent surgical connection between an artery and a vein. Fistulas are used for dialysis procedures and must never be used for venipunctures due to the possibility of infection.

4. **Do not label the tubes prior to the venipuncture.**
5. **Do not leave the patient's room before labeling the tubes.**
6. **Do not dismiss an outpatient before labeling the tubes.**
7. **Do not label tubes using a pencil; black ink should be used.**
8. **Do not leave the patient until you checked and ensure that the bleeding has stopped.**

Routine Venipuncture
1) **Verify the requisition for the tests.**
2) Identify the patient: check the patient's ID number and have him/her state his/her name.
3) **Identify yourself to the patient, explain the procedure, and secure his/her consent.**
4) **Palpate the veins in the antecubital fossa using your index finger.**
5) **Gather the necessary equipment.**
6) Wash hands; put on gloves.
7) **Tie on the tourniquet; it should be applied 3-4 inches above the site where the venipuncture will be made. Ask the patient to make a fist or open and close his/her hand to help engorge the vein.**
8) **Palpate the vein while looking for the straightest point. Cleanse the area using a circular motion starting at the inside of the venipuncture site.**

9) Assemble the needle and tube holder while the alcohol is drying. Uncap the needle and examine it for defects such as blunted or barbed point.
10) Hold the patient's arm, by placing four fingers under the forearm and your thumb below the antecubital area slightly pulling the skin back to anchor the vein.
11) With the bevel facing upward, insert the needle at an angle of 15-30 degrees.
12) Once the needle is inside the vein (you will feel a "give" as the vein is entered), push the collection tube into the holder to puncture the tube stopper with the back-end of the needle.
13) Release the tourniquet once blood flow has begun. The tourniquet should not be left on for more than one (1) minute in order to prevent hemoconcentration.
14) Fill the needed tubes, according to the order of draw.
15) Pull out collection tube from the holder.
16) Place folded gauze over the venipuncture site and withdraw the needle. Then apply pressure until bleeding stops. This is done to prevent hematoma. Do not ask the patient to bend the arm as it does not offer enough pressure.
17) Discard needle into the biohazards sharp container.
18) Label each collected specimen, writing the patient's name and ID number, the time and date of collection, and your initials.
19) Place labeled tubes inside the biohazards transport bag.
20) Before leaving, check the venipuncture site. If it is still bleeding, apply pressure for another 2 minutes. If after this time, it is still bleeding, continue to apply pressure for another 3 minutes. If bleeding persists after a total of 8 minutes of applying pressure, call for help.
21) At any point when the bleeding stops, an adhesive bandage is applied over a folded gauze square. The patient should be instructed to remove the bandage within an hour.
22) Clean up everything and dispose of waste properly.
23) Leave the patient's call light within his/her reach.
24) Remove the gloves, wash your hands, say good-bye to the patient and inform him/her that his/her physician will deliver the results.

Little attention is often given to these steps that are necessary for collecting a blood specimen. Our state-of-the-art sophisticated laboratory technology is often riddled with errors because of misidentification and poor sample collection techniques. All of the steps must be followed without deviation.

Order of Draw
Often requests are for more than one test to be performed; and as such, more than one collection tube needs to be drawn. The correct order of draw is:

- Blood Cultures
- Light Blue top tubes
- Serum or non-additive tube (Red or Red/Gray top tubes)
- Green top tubes
- Lavender top tubes
- Gray top tubes

To help their students memorize the new order of draw, the staff at Phlebotomy Education LLC in Allen Park MI have put together this simple sentence mnemonic: "BeCause Better Specimens Generate Perfect Goals."

BeCause	=	Blood Cultures
Better	=	Blue
Specimens	=	Serum (Red)
Generate	=	Green
Perfect	=	Purple (Lavender)
Goals	=	Gray

Failure to Obtain Blood

Most venipunctures are routine, but in some instances, complications can arise resulting in failure to obtain blood. The following are some of the common causes:

1. The tube has lost its vacuum. This is may be due to:
    1. A manufacturing defect
    2. Expired tube
    3. A very fine crack in the tube
2. Improperly positioned needle. In many instances, slight movement of the needle can correct this.
    1. The bevel of the needle is resting against the wall of the vein. Slightly rotate the needle.
    2. The needle is not fully in the vein. Slowly advance the needle.
    3. The needle has passed through the vein. Slowly pull back on the vein.
    4. The vein was missed completely. With a gloved finger, gently determine the positions of the vein and the needle, and redirect the needle.
3. Collapsed vein. This may be due to excessive pull from the vacuum tube; use of a smaller vacuum tube may remedy the situation. If it does not, remove the tourniquet, withdraw the needle, and select another vein preferably using either a syringe or butterfly.

Complications Associated with Phlebotomy

1. **Hematoma:** The most common complication of phlebotomy procedure. This indicates that blood has accumulated in the tissue surrounding the vein. The two most common causes are the needle going through the vein, and/or failure to apply enough pressure on the site after needle withdrawal.
2. **Hemoconcentration:** The increase in proportion of formed elements to plasma caused by the tourniquet being left on too long. (More than two (2) minutes)
3. **Phlebitis:** Inflammation of a vein as a result of repeated venipuncture on that vein.
4. **Petechiae:** These are tiny non-raised red spots that appear on the skin from rupturing of the capillaries due to the tourniquet being left on too long or too tight.
5. **Thrombus:** This is a blood clot usually a consequence of insufficient pressure applied after the withdrawal of the needle.
6. **Thrombophlebitis:** Inflammation of a vein with formation of a clot

7. **Septicemia:** This is a systemic infection associated with the presence of pathogenic organism introduced during a venipuncture.
8. **Trauma:** This is an injury to underlying tissues caused by probing of the needle.

Special Venipuncture
Some venipunctures are done using special collecting or handling procedures specific to the test being requested. Some require patient preparation such as fasting, while some needs to be collected at a specific time. Still, others may need special handling such as protection from light.

Fasting Specimens
This requires collection of blood while the patient is in the basal state, that is, the patient has fasted and refrained from strenuous exercise for 12 hours prior to the drawing. It is the Certified Phlebotomy Technicians responsibility to verify if the patient indeed, has been fasting for the required time.

Timed Specimens
They are often used to monitor the level of a specific substance or condition in the patient. Blood is drawn at specific times for different reasons. They are:
- To measure blood levels of substances exhibiting diurnal variation. (e.g., cortisol hormone)
- To determine blood levels of medications. (e.g., digoxin for cardiovascular disease)
- To monitor changes in a patient's condition. (e.g., steady decrease in hemoglobin level)

Two-Hour Postprandial Test
This test is used to evaluate diabetes mellitus. Fasting glucose level is compared with the level 2 hours after eating a full meal or ingesting a measured amount of glucose.

Oral Glucose Tolerance Test (OGTT)
This test is used to diagnose diabetes mellitus and evaluate patients with frequent low blood sugar. 3-hour OGTT is used to test hyperglycemia (abnormally high blood sugar level) and diagnose diabetes mellitus. 5-hour OGTT is used to evaluate hypoglycemia (abnormally low blood sugar level) for disorders of carbohydrate metabolism. OGTT are scheduled to begin between 0700 and 0900.

Therapeutic Drug Monitoring
This test is used to monitor the blood levels of certain medication to ensure patient safety and also maintain a plasma level. Blood is drawn to coincide with the trough (lowest blood level) or the peak level (highest blood level). Trough levels are collected 30 minutes before the scheduled dose. Time for collecting peak level will vary depending on the medication, patient's metabolism, and the route of administration (I.V., I.M., or oral).

Blood Cultures (BC)
They are ordered to detect presence of microorganisms in the patient's blood. The patient will usually have chills and fever of unknown origin (FUO), indicating the possible presence of pathogenic microorganisms in the blood (septicemia). Blood cultures are usually ordered STAT or as timed specimen, and collection requires strict aseptic technique.

PKU
This test is ordered for infants to detect phenylketonuria, a genetic disease that causes mental retardation and brain damage. Test is done on blood from newborn's heel or on urine.

Special Specimen Handling

Cold Agglutinins
Cold agglutinins are antibodies produced in response to Mycoplasma pneumoniae infection (atypical pneumonia). The antibodies formed may attach to red blood cells at temperatures below body temperature, and as such, the specimen must be kept warm until the serum is separated from the cells. Blood is collected in red-topped tubes pre-warmed in the incubator at 37 degrees Celsius for 30 minutes.

Chilled specimens
Some tests require that the specimen collected be chilled immediately after collection in crushed ice or ice and water mixture. Likewise, the specimen must be immediately transported to the laboratory for processing. Some of the tests that require chilled specimen are: arterial blood gases, ammonia, lactic acid, pyruvate, ACTH, gastrin, and parathyroid hormone.

Light-sensitive specimens
Specimens are protected from light by wrapping the tubes in aluminum foil immediately after they are drawn. Exposure to light could alter the test results for: Bilirubin, beta-carotene, Vitamins A & B6, and porphyrins.

Dermal Punctures (Microcapillary collection)
When venipuncture is inadvisable, it is possible to perform a majority of laboratory tests on micro samples obtained by dermal (skin) puncture, with the exception of ESR, blood cultures and other tests that require a large amount of serum. Dermal puncture may be done on both pediatric and adult patients.

Punctures should never be performed with a surgical blade or hypodermic needle because they can be difficult to control. Deep penetration into the skin can cause serious injury such as osteomyelitis (inflammation of the bone and bone marrow). A lancet should be used, which delivers a pre-determined depth that can range from 0.85mm for infants to 3.0 mm for adults.

Site selection for dermal puncture
Infants:
The heel is used for dermal punctures on infants less than 1 year of age. Areas recommended are the medial and lateral areas of the plantar surface of the foot. These are determined by drawing imaginary lines medially extending from the middle of the great toe to the heel and laterally from the middle of the fourth and fifth toes to the heel.

The American Academy of Pediatrics recommends that heel punctures for infants not exceed 2.0mm. Observe the following precautions when performing dermal puncture:
- do not puncture deeper than 2.0mm
- do not perform dermal punctures on previous puncture sites
- do not use the back of the heel or arch of the foot.
- use the medial and lateral areas of the plantar surface of the heel

Older children and Adults
The distal segment of the third or fourth finger of the non-dominant hand is the recommended site. Puncture is made in the fleshy portion of the finger slightly to the side of the center perpendicular to the lines of the fingerprint.

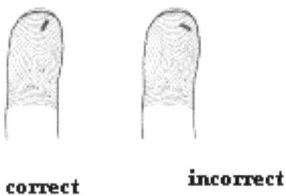

correct   incorrect

Dermal puncture procedure
1. Identify the patient
2. Assemble equipment
3. Warm the site: this is an essential part of the procedure when collecting specimens for pH or blood gases. Warming the site can increase the blood flow up to seven times the normal amount. The specimen is referred to as arterialized specimen because of the increase arterial flow to the area. This is accomplished by warming the site for a minimum of three minutes with a warm moistened towel (no greater than 108 F), or with a commercial warming device.
4. Clean the site: Use 70% isopropyl alcohol. Allow the site to dry for maximum antiseptic action. Alcohol residue can cause hemolysis of the red blood cells and may interfere with glucose testing. Povidone- iodine (Betadine) is not used for cleaning the site because it interferes with several tests like bilirubin, uric acid, phosphorous, and potassium.
5. Prepare the puncture device
6. Perform the dermal puncture

Order of draw for capillary specimens
1. Lavender tube
2. Tubes with other additives
3. Tubes without additives

Microsamples are labeled with the same information required for venipuncture specimens.

Test Tubes, Additives and Tests

◊ **Lavender top tube -**
Contains the anticoagulant ethylenediaminetetraacetic acid (EDTA). EDTA inhibits coagulation by binding to calcium present in the specimen. The tubes must be filled at least two-thirds full and inverted eight times.

Common tests: CBC (Complete Blood Count); Includes: RBC count, WBC count and Platelet count; WBC differential count; Hemoglobin and Hematocrit determinations; ESR (Erythrocyte Sedimentation Rate); Sickle Cell Screening

◊ **Light-Blue top tube -**
Contains the anticoagulant Sodium Citrate, which also prevents coagulation by binding to calcium in the specimen. Sodium citrate is the anticoagulant used for coagulation studies because it preserves the coagulation factors. The tube must be filled completely to maintain the ratio of nine parts blood to one part sodium citrate, and should be inverted three to four times.

Common tests: Coagulation Studies- Prothrombin Time (PT) – evaluates the extrinsic; system of the coagulation cascade and monitors; Coumadin therapy; Activated Partial Thromboplastin Time (APTT, PTT) - Evaluates the intrinsic system of the coagulation cascade and monitors Heparin therapy. Fibrinogen Degradation Products (FDP) Thrombin Time (TT); Factor assays, Bleeding Time (BT)

◊ **Green top tube -**
Contains the anticoagulant Heparin combined with sodium, lithium, or ammonium ion. Heparin works by inhibiting thrombin in the coagulation cascade. It is not used for hematology because heparin interferes with the Wright's stained blood smear. This tube should be inverted eight times.

Common tests: Chemistry tests: performed on plasma such as Ammonia, carboxyhemoglobin & STAT electrolytes.

◊ **Gray top tube –**
Contains additives and anticoagulants. All gray top tubes contain glucose preservative (antiglycolytic agent): sodium fluoride- preserves glucose for 3days; or lithium iodoacetate- preserves glucose for 24 hours. May also contain the anticoagulant potassium oxalate, which prevents clotting by binding calcium. This tube should be inverted eight times.

Common tests: Fasting blood sugar (FBS); Glucose tolerance test (GTT); Blood alcohol levels; Lactic acid measurement

- ◊ **Red/Gray (speckled) top tube -**
  Also called tiger-top tube and serum separator tubes (SST). Contain clot activators: glass particles, silica and celite which hastens clot formation, and thixotropic gel, a serum separator which when centrifuged forms a barrier between the serum and the cells preventing contamination of the serum with cellular elements. Tubes must be inverted five times.

  Common tests: Most chemistry tests

- ◊ **Red top tube -**
  Also known as plain vacuum tube and contains no additive or anticoagulant. Collected blood clots by normal coagulation process in 30-60 minutes. There is no need to invert the tube after collection.

  Common tests – Serum chemistry tests; Serology tests; Blood bank (glass only)

- ◊ **Yellow top tube -** (sterile)
  Contains the anticoagulant sodium polyanetholesulfonate (SPS). These are used to collect specimens to be cultured for the presence of microorganisms. The SPS aids in the recovery of microorganisms by inhibiting the actions of complement, phagocytes, and certain antibiotics. These tubes should be inverted eight times.

Quality Control (QC)

The primary purpose of a quality control program is to provide reliable data about the patient's health status by ensuring the accuracy of test results while detecting and eliminating errors.

At least once a day, when tests are performed, check tests through control specimens must also be done to make sure the results are reliable and valid. In some laboratories, controls are done with every batch of tests. Normal, and abnormal (both in low ranges and high ranges) controls maybe performed with the testing.

Standards
This is a substance of known value essentially free of impurities and have close to a "true" value. Although too expensive for daily use in the laboratory, they serve as excellent reference standards to ensure accuracy of testing.

Proficiency Testing Systems
Proficiency testing systems are a requirement for laboratories. State, local or private agencies send sera to the laboratories for testing, the results of which are sent back to the agencies. Test results are compared with those of other participating laboratories and printed summaries are provided to them. When test results do not compare with the other laboratories, this is an indication for a need for improvements. If a laboratory repeatedly fails in the testing, state regulatory agencies may not allow that laboratory to perform a particular test until corrective measures are instituted.

Maintenance Programs
Maintenance schedule for all laboratory instruments must be in place so that they stay in correct working condition. Maintenance activities include regular calibrating of instruments, checking refrigerator and freezer temperature, water purity testing to name a few.

Clinical Laboratory Sections
The medical laboratory is an area in a healthcare facility where body fluids, cells, and tissues are analyzed. Size and setup can vary; however, most full-function clinical laboratories have four sections: clinical chemistry, hematology, microbiology, and blood bank.

Hematology Section
This department deals with the various components of the blood: white blood cells, red blood cells, platelets. Tests performed may be quantitative which involve actual number counts. Complete blood count is the most common test performed. Tests maybe qualitative which focus on the quality or characteristics such as size, shape and maturity of the cells. Other procedures include: retic count, sed rate, and red cells indices.

Coagulation frequently is a subsection in this department. Coagulation tests are done to determine discrepancies in the clotting mechanism, the most common of which are prothrombin time and activated partial thromboplastin time.

Chemistry Section
The most automated section in the laboratory. This section is divided into several areas:
1. **Electrophoresis** – analyzes chemical components of blood such as hemoglobin and serum, urine and cerebrospinal fluid, based on the differences in electrical charge.
2. **Toxicology** - analyzes plasma levels of drugs and poisons.
3. **Immunochemistry** – This section uses techniques such as radio immunoassay (RIA) and enzyme immunoassay to detect and measure substances such as hormones, enzymes, and drugs.

Some tests in the chemistry section are ordered by profiles, which are groups of tests ordered by a physician to evaluate the status of an organ, body system or general health of the patient. Examples of these profiles are:
- ◊ Liver profile: tests may include ALP, AST, ALT, GGT and Bilirubin
- ◊ Coronary risk profile: tests may include Cholesterol, Triglycerides, HDL, LDL

Blood Bank Section
This is the section where blood is collected, stored and prepared for transfusion. Strict adherence to procedures for patient identification and specimen handling is a must to ensure patient safety. Blood collected may be separated into components: packed cells, platelets, fresh frozen plasma, and cryoprecipitate.

Specimen Requirements
Tests done in the blood bank require a red top (plain) tube or a lavender or pink top tube. Specimens must have the following identification information:
1. Patient's full name and date of birth
2. Patient's hospital identification number (SSN for outpatients)
3. Date and time of collection
4. Phlebotomist's initials

The most common testing done includes ABO and Rh typing, the antibody screen (indirect antibody test), and crossmatch. Other tests may include antibody panel testing, test for hemolytic disease of the newborn, hemolytic transfusion reactions, and direct antiglobulin test.

Exact procedures for the proper identification of a patient, a patient's sample, and a donor's blood is established to guard against clerical errors which will cause transfusion accidents.

Blood type

ABO Blood Group System: The surface of RBCs contains antigens that determine the blood group and blood type of the patient. There are four ABO blood groups based on the antigens present. Group A blood has "A" antigen, group B has "B" antigen, group AB has both "A" and "B" antigens, and group O has neither "A" nor "B" antigen on the cell membrane. Groups O and A are the most common and group AB is the least common blood group.

ABO Blood Group System

Blood Type	RBC Antigen	Plasma Antibodies
A	A	Anti-B
B	B	Anti-A
AB	A and B	neither Anti-A nor Anti-B
O	either	Anti-A and Anti-B

Rh Blood Group System

The presence or absence of the "D" antigen (also known as the Rh factor) on the RBC membrane determines whether a person is Rh positive or negative. Hence, a individual whose RBCs have the D antigen are Rh positive (Rh+), and an individual whose RBCs lack the D antigen are Rh negative (Rh -). The D antigen is present in approximately 85% of the population.

Serology (Immunology) Section

Performs tests to evaluate the patient's immune response through the production of antibodies. This section uses serum to analyze presence of antibodies to bacteria, viruses, fungi, parasites and antibodies against the body's own substances (autoimmunity).

Microbiology Section

Culture and sensitivity is the primary test done to detect the presence and identify the microorganisms in body fluids and tissues. Subsections are:
1. Bacteriology – the study of bacteria
2. Parasitology – the study of parasites
3. Mycology - the study of fungi
4. Virology – the study of viruses

Urinalysis Section

This department performs physical, chemical, and microscopic examination of urine. The physical examination assesses the color, clarity, and specific gravity of the specimen. Chemical evaluation is done using chemical reagent strips to screen for substances such as sugar and protein. Microscopic examination is done to detect presence of blood cells, bacteria and other substances. Requested cultures are sent the microbiology department.

The Microscope
One of the most commonly used instruments in the medical laboratory is the compound microscope also known as the bright-field microscope. It has two different lenses and light passes through the specimen and lenses to the observer's eye. Lens on the eyepiece (ocular) compounds or increases the magnification produced of an image by the other lens (objective). Magnification is determined by multiplying the magnifying power of the ocular lens (10X) by the magnifying power of the objective lens (10X, 40X, 100X). The objectives are mounted on a nosepiece which pivots to allow the lenses to rotate. Objective lenses are rated according to focal length (usually, 16-mm, 4-mm, and 1.8-mm) which is the distance from the object examined to the center of the lens. The greater the magnification of the lens, the lesser is the distance between the bottom of the lens and the material viewed.

> **Low power objective** (16-mm, 10X)
> This allows the item being viewed to be magnified ten times larger than life. This magnification multiplied with the magnification of the ocular lens allows us to see microscopically one hundred times the normal size (10X x 10X = 100X). This is used for light adjustment, for initial focusing and scanning a subject (e.g. observing the morphology of microorganisms).
>
> **High power objective** (4-mm, 40X)
> By combining the ten-power (10X) ocular lens with the magnification power of forty times life40X), the magnification vision is increased to four hundred times the normal size (10X x 40X = 400X). This is used to view urinary sediments in detail, KOH prep for fungi, and wet mounts for parasites.
>
> **Oil immersion objective** (1.8-mm, 100X)
> This objective enables us to reach a possible total magnification of one thousand times normal life size by multiplying the ocular lens magnification (10X) by one hundred (100X), (10X x 100X = 1,000X). Since more light is needed to actually see this amount of magnification, the lens is immersed in oil. Oil slows down
>
> The speed at which light travels preventing the scattering or loss of light rays which naturally occurs when light travels through air. Consequently, the efficiency of the magnification is increased.
>
> This objective is used for observing bacteria, for WBC differential count and RBC morphology

Understanding Laboratory Measurements

Basic Units of the System

Meter
The meter is the basic unit of length. A meter is 39.37 inches long. A decimeter would be 3.94 inches long. A centimeter would be about 0.39 inches long, and a millimeter would be about 0.04 inches in length. One thousand meters would equal 1 km. Meters are often used in laboratory reports, charts, and other data requiring linear measurements. For instance, a laboratory procedure might require you to "connect flasks using 0.3 meters of rubber tubing;" this would mean that you must use 12 inches of tubing.

Liter

The liter is the basic unit of capacity or volume. This measure tells us how much space an item occupies. The standard unit for capacity in the International System is expressed in terms of multiples or decimal fractions of the cubic meter. In the laboratory, this unit is too large for everyday use; thus the cubic decimeter is used. The liter is accepted as a general designation for 1 cubic decimeter. The liter is used most frequently in the United States by the beverage industry. We are all familiar with the 2-liter soft drink container. A liter is slightly more than 1 qt and is equal to 1000 mL, or the capacity occupied by 2.2 lb of distilled water at 39.2*C.

Gram

The gram is the basic unit of weight or mass. A measure of weight tells how heavy an item is. One thousand cubic centimeters, the equivalent of 1 cubic decimeter, have the capacity of 1 L and weigh 1000 gm or 1 kg. The kilogram is the standard unit of weight and is equivalent to approximately 2.2 lb in the English system of measurement. In the clinical laboratory, the gram (0.001 kg) is used more frequently than is the kilogram. A gram is the weight of 1 cubic centimeter of distilled water at a temperature of 39.2*C.

Metric Abbreviations

Metric Unit	Abbreviation	Meter	Liter	Gram
Meter	M(m)			
Liter	L (l)			
Gram	g or gm			
Kilo	k	km	kL	kg
Hecto	h	hm	hL	hg
Deca	da	dam	daL	dag
Deci	d	dm	mL	dg
Centi	c	cm	cL	cg
Milli	m	mm	mL	mg
Micro	u	um	uL	ug

Commonly Used Metric Prefixes

Kilo = 1000.00 (One-thousand)
Deci = 0.1 (one-tenth)
Centi = 0.01 (one-hundredth)
Milli = 0.001 (one-thousandth)
Micro = 0.000,001 (one millionth)
Nano = 0.000,000,001 (one billionth)

Solutions and Dilutions

It is necessary to make dilutions in the laboratory frequently. For example, blood, serum, or plasma is diluted to produce color reactions that can be used in determining test results. When blood cell counts are done manually, it is necessary to make a dilution before these cells can be counted under the microscope.

Today, most solutions are commercially prepared and come to the laboratory in a ready-to use package. You know that a 10% bleach solution is the solution of choice in cleaning areas where there is the possibility of body fluid contamination. There will be a time that you will need to prepare a solution of certain strength from a given solution of another strength. Whenever solution preparation is required, accuracy is essential. When preparing a solution, it must be accomplished to exact specifications.

Preparing Solutions and Dilutions
Whenever a dilution is to be prepared, the formula is as follows:

$$\frac{\text{Desired strength}}{\text{Available strength}} = \frac{X \text{ (amount needed)}}{\text{amount available}}$$

Arterial Blood Gas Studies
Arterial blood gas studies (ABGs) are valuable tools in the treatment of critically ill patients. As the name suggests, ABGs are one of the few clinical laboratory procedures performed on arterial blood. Arterial blood gas analyzers quantitate ABG components using special electrodes. ABGs help assess a patient's ventilation, oxygenation, and acid-base balance. ABGs are also used to monitor the condition of critically ill patients, to diagnose electrolyte imbalances, to monitor oxygen flow rates, and to complement other pulmonary function studies. It should be remembered that any arterial puncture should not be attempted by anyone who is not trained and licensed to perform this procedure.

The Gram Stain
The Gram Stain is used to classify bacteria on the basis of their form, size, cellular morphology, and Gram Stain reaction. It is a critical test for the rapid presumptive identification of infectious agents, and it also is a means by which the quality of clinical specimen can be evaluated.

When exposed to the Gram Stain, bacteria stain either gram-positive (deep violet) or gram-negative (light to dark red) on the basis of differences in cell wall composition and structure. Gram-positive bacteria have a thick peptidoglycan layer and large amounts of teichoic acids. This combination prevents them from being affected by alcohol decolorization; therefore, they retain the initial stain of crystal violet, which imparts a deep violet color. Gram-negative cell walls have a single peptidoglycan layer attached to a symmetric, lipoplysaccharide, phospholipid, bilayered, outer membrane interspersed with protein. The outer membrane is damaged by the alcohol decolorizer, allowing the crystal violet iodine complex to leak out and be replaced by the Sefranin counterstain (red). The Gram stain can be affected by many factors, including culturing, age, antibiotics, the medium in which the bacteria is growing, incubation, atmosphere, phagocytosis, and staining technique.

The most important bacterial property for classification purposes is a simple procedure that employs the aniline dye, crystal violet. The cell wall structure appears to be the determining factor by which bacteria react to the Gram stain.

1. Gram-positive bacteria: are bacteria that take up and retain the crystal violet and resist alcohol decoloration. They appear blue to black.
2. Gram-negative bacteria: are bacteria that are decolorized completely by ethanol and take up safranin counterstain. They appear red.

Gram staining is only a first step. Biochemical tests may have to be done before a final diagnosis is made. However, therapeutic decisions can be made based on this test.

The Gram staining procedure consists of the following sequence:
1. Dye – crystal violet
2. Mordant – Gram's iodine
3. Decolorizer – 95% ethyl alcohol/acetone mixture
4. Counterstain – safranin stain

Smear Preparation
Proper smear preparation will produce a thin monolayer of organisms for easy visualization but will be thick enough to reveal characteristic arrangements of the bacteria. Always wear latex gloves and a laboratory coat and follow all other universal precautions when handling clinical specimens.

Pre-cleaned, glass slides with frosted ends should be used for the smear. The frosted ends are desirable as they allow accurate labeling and convenient handling. Frequently, a direct smear is prepared from the swab used to obtain the sample. A smear can be from any body opening, including the genitals or wounds (such as surgical sites, bites, cuts, or body ulcers). The best process is to obtain two swabs, one for the culture and one for the smear. If this is the case, the specimen is cultured first. Then, before the thioglycolate tube is inoculated, the smear is prepared. The danger in using one swab is that the target area may be missed, thus invalidating the entire testing process. You will want to check laboratory protocols for smear preparation to determine the exact procedure for obtaining a smear specimen.

Smearing and Fixation Technique
To prepare the smear, gently roll the swab across the slide, in one direction, leaving **a thin** film of specimen material on the slide. Specimens not received on swabs can be spread over a large area by using sterile swabs or a heat-sterilized wire loop to form a thin film on the slide. Extremely thick specimens can be placed on one slide, covered with a second slide, and pulled apart. The excess on the edge of the slide can be removed using a disinfectant-soaked paper towel. The smearing and fixation technique must be done in a bio safety cabinet.

Smears should be air-dried on a flat surface or on an electric slide warmer heated to 60 degrees Centigrade. The slide is placed on the supporting rods of the stain rack and then fixed by covering the slide with methanol for 1 minute. The residual methanol is then drained off without rinsing and is allowed to air-dry again. The slide is then ready to stain. Do no heat-fix the slide before staining. Methanol fixation is preferred over the old standard of heat-fixing smears because it prevents lysis of red blood cells (RBCs), gives a cleaner background, does not affect bacterial morphology, and is safer.

Staining Bacteria
The staining procedure involves the sequential application of primary stain mordant, decolorizer, and counterstain to a bacterial smear. The organisms according to the chemical composition of the cell walls take up the stains differently. A fixed smear is placed on a staining rack and the primary stain crystal violet is poured onto one end of the smear until the whole side is covered. The stain is allowed to remain in one place for 30 seconds.

Staining of Blood Smears

The stain commonly used for examination of blood cells is called polychromatic because they contain dyes that will stain various cell components different colors. These stains usually contain methylene blue, a blue stain, and eosin, a re-orange stain. These stains are attracted to different parts of the cell. Thus, the cells and their structures can be more easily visualized and differentiated. The most commonly used differential bloodstain is Wright's Stain.

Semi-automated slide stainers are frequently used in large laboratories. These machines are capable of staining a large number of blood smears with consistency and reliability. Small laboratories generally use a manual quick stain method.

Urinalysis

Components of the urinary system
This system consists of two kidneys, two ureters, urinary bladder, and a urethra.

The kidney is the primary organ of the urinary system. The two kidneys are bean-shaped organs located on each side of the body behind the peritoneum on the back wall of the abdominal cavity. In cross-section, each kidney has an outer region, the renal cortex, and an inner region, the renal medulla. Urine flows from the collecting ducts to the renal pelvis and through the ureter into the bladder.

The kidneys' functions are: to remove metabolic waste from the blood stream, maintain the body's acid-base balance and regulate body hydration. Urea, a nitrogenous product of protein metabolism, is the major waste product removed by the kidney. The kidney's ability to reabsorb into the blood stream water and chemicals previously filtered from the blood allows it to regulate the acid-base and fluid balance of the body.

Hormones are also produced such as renin which controls blood pressure and erythropoietin which stimulates the production of red blood cells.

The two ureters are muscular tubes that carry urine from the kidney to the bladder. The bladder is an expandable sac located in the pelvis; it stores the urine formed by the filtration of blood in the glomerulus of the nephron. The urethra is the tube extending from the bladder to the external opening.

Collecting the Urine Specimen
The manner in which the specimen is collected depends on the test to be performed. In the medical office, the collection, processing, and/or transport of most specimens can be accomplished without complication. Patient education is the responsibility of the medical assistant, and collecting a urine specimen requires clear and concise instructions.

General Instructions for Urine Collection
Urine specimens may be collected in the medical office or at home. In either situation, it is important to follow appropriate procedures for specimen collection and processing.

Instructions for Urine Collection

1. Carefully label all specimens. Do not apply the label to the container lid, but place the label on the container itself. Use an indelible marker or make sure that the label will adhere to the container at refrigerated temperatures. On the label, record the patient's name, the date and time of collection, and the type of specimen. Add the physician's name if the specimen is to be sent to a central laboratory facility opening that is 2 inches in diameter. If the specimen is to be obtained from a pediatric patient, the container may be slightly smaller. If the specimen is to be transported, be sure it has a screw-type lid.
2. If a bacterial culture is ordered, make sure a sterile container is available. If this is the case, the specimen may have to be obtained through catheterization.
3. Advise female patients, with the consent of the physician, that the collection of a urine specimen should be avoided, if possible, during their menstrual cycle and for several days before and after, as the specimen may be contaminated with blood.
4. If the analyte is unstable or if the testing is delayed, you may add preservatives to the specimen. Check your laboratory's procedure manual or the procedural manual provided by the referral laboratory to determine the proper preservative for each test. Remember that the preservative must not interfere with the test procedure or results. Always not on the specimen the type and amount of preservative added.

Types of Specimen Collection

First Morning Sample

A first morning sample is the type of specimen most commonly used for routine urinalysis. Because the concentration of urine varies throughout the day, it is usually easiest to identify abnormalities in a relatively concentrated specimen. The first morning specimen may also be called an early morning specimen, as it represents the urine formed over approximately an 8-hour period.

Because it is impractical to collect a first morning specimen in the medical office, the patient must be instructed in the proper collection technique for a clean-catch or mid-stream urine sample. The specimen can then be collected at home and brought to the office. Be certain that the patient knows to refrigerate the specimen until it is transported to the office. The laboratory should supply the container, as a container from home may not be properly washed and rinsed prior to use. When the specimen is delivered to the office or laboratory, the medical assistant should check it for proper labeling and perform the required test(s) immediately. If that is not possible, the specimen may be refrigerated until testing can be done.

Mid-Stream Specimen

A mid-stream urine specimen is one that is collected not at the beginning or end of voiding, but in the middle of urination. The patient is instructed to void the first one third of the urine into the toilet. At the point, the patient stops urine flow, places the specimen container into position, and voids the next one third of the urine into the container. Once the specimen is collected, the patient can then finish emptying the bladder into the toilet. The specimen volume should be at least 25 mL of urine. A mid-stream specimen is thought to be a better representative of the contents of the bladder.

Clean-Catch Specimen

Most laboratories prefer a clean-catch, mid-stream specimen for testing, as it provides the clearest, most accurate results. If the urine specimen is to be tested for bacteria or antibiotic sensitivity and a catheterized specimen is not required, a clean-catch sample will be needed. Collecting this sample requires special cleaning of the external genitalia. Because most patients are not familiar with aseptic technique, they must be carefully instructed on the procedure. In the case of a disabled or elderly individual, assistance may be needed in obtaining the specimen.

Urine composition
Urine formed by a healthy kidney is approximately 96% water and 4% dissolved substances consisting mainly of urea (a nitrogenous product of protein metabolism), sodium chloride, sulfates and phosphates. Abnormal constituents include RBCs and WBCs, fat, glucose, casts, bile, acetone, and hemoglobin. Other substances may be present in small quantities like calcium, hormones, proteins, fatty acids, and metals.

Urine Output
The actual amount of urinary output is dependent upon the body's state of hydration and normally averages 1200-1500ml every 24 hours. Decreased urinary output is termed oliguria. Increased output is called polyuria, and little or no urine output is known as anuria.

Routine Urinalysis
Examination of the urine is a diagnostic tool to detect or monitor certain conditions. It is often requested because urine is easily obtained and much information about the body can be had from the result of the test.

Examination of Urine
The routine urinalysis procedure is composed of three parts:
1. physical examination
2. chemical examination
3. microscopic examination

Physical examination of urine
This consists of:
1. Assessing the volume of the urine specimen to determine if it
2. Is adequate for testing.
3. Observing the color and appearance (or character) of the
4. specimen
5. Noting the odor.
6. Measuring the specific gravity.

Chemical examination of urine
This involves chemical evaluation of the contents of the urine which can be qualitative or quantitative. The chemical testing may involve examination of the following:
7. pH
8. Glucose
9. Ketone
10. Protein
11. Blood
12. Bilirubin
13. Urobilinogen
14. Nitrite
15. Leukocyte esterase

Microscopic examination of the urine
This is the microscopic examination done on urine sediment obtained by centrifugation of 10 to 15ml of urine. The identification and enumeration of the urinary sediment constituents require that only highly skilled and qualified individuals undertake the microscopic examination.

Specific Gravity
The specific gravity of urine is the ratio of the weight of a given volume of urine to the weight of the same volume of distilled water at a constant temperature. Specific gravity is the most convenient way of measuring the kidneys' ability to concentrate and dilute. An abnormality in the ability of the kidney to concentrate or dilute urine is an indication of renal disease or hormonal deficiency.

During a 24-hour period, normal adults with normal diets and normal fluid intake produce urine with a specific gravity of between 1.015 and 1.025. The normal range of urine specific gravity for a random collection is 1.005 to 1.030.

Urinary pH
The pH, or the percentage of hydrogen ion concentration of a solution, is a reflection of the acidity or alkaline of a solution. A pH of 7.0 is considered to be neutral. The pH of distilled water is 7.0. A pH of 0 to 7.0 is considered to be acidic, whereas a pH of 7 to 14 is considered to be alkaline or basic.

Normal, freshly voided urine will usually have a pH of 4.5 to 8.0. Within this range, the urine pH of most healthy patients is around 6.0.

Urinary Glucose
Glucose is the sugar typically found in urine. Other sugars, such as lactose, fructose, galactose, and pentose, may be detected in urine under specific circumstances. Glucose is present in urine when the blood glucose level exceeds the renal threshold. Glycosuria is the presence of glucose in the urine.

Patients with diabetes mellitus have glycosuria, along with polynuria and thirst. The reagent strip test for glucose relies on enzymatic tests that are specific for glucose. A common reagent strip urinary glucose enzymatic method uses glucose oxidase. The glucose oxidase reacts specifically with glucose. Sugars, such as lactose, fructose, and others, are not detected by the glucose oxidase method. A copper reaction test is a commonly used confirmatory and screening test for glucose and other reducing substances in urine. Copper reduction tests are used in pediatric patients to detect increased levels of glucose that may not be detected by the specific enzymatic test found on most reagent strips.

Urinary Bacteria
Enteric gram-negative bacteria that are always nitrite positive can convert urinary nitrate to nitrite. A positive nitrite test is an indication that a significant number of bacteria are present in the urine.

Urinary Leukocytes

The presence of increased numbers of leukocytes or white blood cells in the urine is an indicator of bacteriuria or urinary tract infection (UTI). Granulocytic leukocytes release esterase when the cells lyse. Testing for leukocyte esterase by the reagent strip method is used in tandem with the microscopic examination of urine sediment for the diagnosis of bacteriuria or UTI.

A positive test by the reagent strip method is indicated by a purple color. The greater the amount of leukocytes/esterase present, the greater the intensity of the purple color. Bacterial culture and sensitivity testing best confirm UTI's. A clean-catch mid-stream urine sample is usually required for any bacterial culture. For this reason, it is ALWAYS wise to collect a clean-catch urine specimen; do not dispose of the specimen until the physician directs you to do so.

Specialized Urine Tests/Urinary Pregnancy Testing

Probably the most common specialized urine test is the pregnancy test. Human chorionic gonadotropin (hCG), also known as uterine chorionic gonadotropin (UCG), is produced in the placenta and is detectable in the blood and urine early in the gestation period. HCG is not normally found in the urine of young, healthy, non-pregnant women. Because of hCG's early appearance during gestation, increased levels of hCG are a natural marker for pregnancy.

Legal Considerations

Informed consent

This is consent given by the patient who is made aware of any procedure to be performed, its risks, expected outcomes, and alternatives.

Patient confidentiality

This is the key concept of HIPAA. All patients have a right to privacy and all information should remain privileged. Discuss patient information only with the patient's physician or office personnel that need certain information to do their job. Obtain a signed consent form to release medical information to the insurance company or other individual.

Negligence

This is the failure to exercise the standard of care that a reasonable person would give under similar circumstances and someone suffers injury because of another's failure to live up to a required duty of care.

The four elements of negligence, (4 Ds), are:
1. Duty: duty of care
2. Derelict: breach of duty of care
3. Direct cause: legally recognizable injury occurs as a result of the breach of duty of care.
4. Damage: wrongful activity must have caused the injury or harm that occurred.

Tort

Is a wrongful act that results in injury to one person by another. Some examples of common torts that can occur in the clinic are the following:

- *Battery* - The basis of tort in this case is the unprivileged touching of one person by another. When a procedure is to be performed on a patient, the patient must give consent in full knowledge of the procedure and the risk it entails (informed consent).
- *Invasion of privacy* – This is the release of medical records without the patient's knowledge and permission.
- *Defamation of character* – This consists of injury to another person's reputation, name, or character through spoken (slander) or written (libel) words.

Good Samaritan Law - This law deals with the rendering of first aid by health care professionals at the scene of an accident or sudden injury. It encourages health care professionals to provide medical care within the scope of their training without fear of being sued for negligence

Needle Stick Prevention Act
OSHA has put into force the Occupational Exposure to Bloodborne Pathogen (BBP) Standard when it was concluded that healthcare employees face a serious health risk as a result of occupational exposure to blood and other body fluids and tissues. The standards outline necessary engineering and work practice controls that OSHA believes will help minimize or eliminate exposure to employees. The standard was revised in 2001 to conform to the Needlestick Safety and Prevention Act passed in November 2000. The act directed OSHA to revise the BBP standard in four key areas:
- Revision and updating of the exposure control plan.
- Solicitation of employee input in selecting engineering and work practice controls.
- Modification of definitions relating to engineering controls (i.e., sharps disposal containers, self-sheathing needles, needleless systems.
- New record keeping requirements.

The employer must establish and maintain a sharps injury log for percutaneous injury from contaminated sharps and it must be done in such a manner to protect the confidentiality of the injured employee.

The sharps injury log must contain, at a minimum:
a. The type and brand of device involved in the incident.
b. The department or work area where the exposure incident occurred.
c. An explanation of how the incident occurred.

APPENDIX A: Patients Bill Of Rights

As a patient in XXX Hospital you have the right, consistent with law, to:

- Receive treatment without discrimination as to race, color, religion, gender, national origin, disability, or source of payment.
- Receive considerate and respectful care in a clean and safe environment free of unnecessary restraints.
- Receive emergency care if you need it.
- Be informed of the name and position of the doctor who will be in charge of your care in the hospital.
- Know the names, positions and functions of any hospital staff involved in your care.
- Receive complete information about your diagnosis, treatment and prognosis.
- Receive all the information that you need to give informed consent for any proposed procedure or treatment. This information shall include the possible risks and benefits of the procedure or treatment.
- Receive all the information you need to give informed consent for an order not to resuscitate. You also have the right to designate an individual to give this consent for you if you are too ill to do so. If you would like additional information, please ask
- Refuse treatment, examination, or observation, if retired or a family member, and be told what effect this may have on your health.
- Refuse to take part in research. In deciding whether or not to participate, you have the right to a full explanation.
- Privacy while in the hospital and confidentiality of all information and records regarding your care.
- Participate in all decisions about your treatment and discharge from the hospital.
- Review your medical record without charge. Obtain a copy of your medical record for which the hospital can charge a reasonable fee. You cannot be denied a copy solely because you cannot afford to pay.
- Receive a bill and explanation of all charges.
- Complain without fears of reprisals about the care and services you are receiving and to have the hospital respond to you; and if requested, a written response. If you are not satisfied with the hospital's response, you can complain to the Patient Representative Office located here in the hospital.
- Receive information about pain and pain relief measures, be involved in pain management plan, and receive a quick response to reports of pain.
- Receive healthcare in an environment that is dedicated to avoiding patient harm and improving patient safety.
- The right to request information about advance directives regarding your decisions about medical care.
- Make known your wishes in regard to anatomical gifts. Your may document your wishes in your health care proxy or on a donor card, available from the hospital.
- Understand and use these rights. If for any reason you do not understand or you need help, the hospital will attempt to provide assistance, including an interpreter.

Patient Responsibilities

Provision of Information: You have the responsibility to provide, to the best of your knowledge, accurate and complete information about present complaints, past illness, hospitalizations, medications, and other matters relating to your health. You have the responsibility to report unexpected changes in your condition to the responsible practitioner. You are responsible for making it known whether you clearly comprehend a contemplated course of action and what is expected of you.

Compliance with Instructions: You are responsible for following the treatment plan recommended by the practitioner primarily responsible for your care. This may include following the instructions of nurses and allied health personnel as they carry out the coordinated plan of care and implement the responsible practitioner's orders, and as they enforce the applicable hospital rules and regulations. You are responsible for keeping appointments and, when you are unable to do so for any reason, for notifying the responsible practitioner or the hospital.
Refusal of Treatment: You are responsible for your actions if you refuse treatment or do not follow the practitioner's instructions.
Hospital Rules and Regulations: You are responsible for following hospital rules and regulation affecting patient care and conduct.
Respect and Consideration: You are responsible for being considerate of the rights of other patients and hospital personnel and for assisting in the control of noise, smoking and the number of visitors. You are responsible for being respectful of the property of other persons and the hospital.

Patient Representative

The Patient Representative's primary assignment is to assist you in exercising your rights as a patient. He/she is also available to act as your advocate and to provide a specific channel through which you can seek solutions to problems, concerns and unmet needs. You may call the Patient Representative at (000)000-0000.

The Patient Bill of Rights for Pain Management

You have the right to:
- Information about pain and pain relief
- A caring staff who believe your reports of pain
- A care staff with concern about your pain
- A quick response when you report your pain

You have the responsibility to:
- Ask for pain relief when your pain first starts
- Help those caring for you to assess your pain
- Tell those caring for you if your pain is not relieved
- Tell those caring for you about any worries that you have about taking pain medications
- Decide if you want your family and/or significant others to aid in your relief of pain

References

1. Ernst, Dennis, J. Applied Phlebotomy. Lippencott Williams & Wilkins.2005
2. Young, Kennedy. Kinn's the Medical Assistant. Elsevier, 2005
3. OSHA Instruction CPL 2-2.44, Occupational Safety and Health Reporter, Bureau of National Affairs Inc. Washington DC
4. McCall, Ruth E., Phlebotomy Essentials. Lippencott Williams & Wilkins
5. Principles of Clinical Electrocardiography, 13th edition, Goldschlager, Nora, MD.; Goldman Mervin J., MD
6. The only EKG Book You'll Ever Need, 4th Edition. Thaler, Malcom S., MD
7. Gray's Anatomy. Gray, Henry. FRS., Carter, HV., MD
8. www.phlebotomy.com
9. www.OSHA.gov
10. http://davidge2.umaryland.edu

Sample Test Questions

1. 1. What is the key concept of HIPAA?
    1. a. Confidentiality/Privacy
    2. b. Insurance verification
    3. c. Patient account receivables
    4. d. Professionalism

2. 2. Which of the following is not part of the vital signs of body function?
    1. a. Temperature
    2. b. Pulse
    3. c. Respiration
    4. d. Weight

3. 3. In the axillary method of measuring temperature, the temperature is taken:
    1. a. In the mouth
    2. b. In the underarm
    3. c. In the rectum
    4. d. In the ear

4. 4. Rectal temperatures should not be taken from which of the following patients:
    1. a. Infants

- 2. b. Patients with heart disease
- 3. c. Patients who have had facial, neck, nose or mouth injuries
- 4. d. All patients can have their temperatures taken rectally

5. 5. The normal pulse of an adult ranges between:
1. a. 20-40 beats per minute
2. b. 60-100 beats per minute
3. c. 100-120 beats per minute
4. d. 120-160 beats per minute

6. 6. The size of the cuff of the sphygmomanometer will depend on:
1. a. The diameter of the limb
2. b. Age of the patient
3. c. The artery being used
4. d. The diagnosis

7. 7. Each of the following factors will give the Medical Assistant an error in blood pressure measurement, except:
1. a. Improper cuff size
2. b. The arm is not at heart level
3. c. The cuff is deflated at 2-3 mmHG per second
4. d. The cuff is re-inflated during the procedure without allowing the arm to rest

8. 8. When the examiner uses the sense of touch to determine the characteristics of an organ system, the examiner is using which principle of physical examination?
1. a. Inspection
2. b. Percussion
3. c. Palpation
4. d. Auscultation

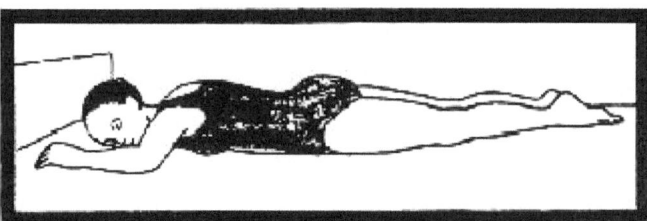

9. 9. The patient above is in which position?
1. a. Semi Fowlers
2. b. Dorsal Recumbent
3. c. Sim's Position
4. d. Prone Position

10. Which method of sterilization is used for instruments that easily corrode?
   a. Chemical sterilization
   b. Dry heat sterilization
   c. Steam sterilization
   d. Gas sterilization

11. Which of the following precautions could be categorized under "Standard Precautions?"
   a. Disposal of all needles and sharp objects in a puncture proof container
   b. Specialized air filters
   c. Sterilization of all instruments
   d. Accurate chart documentation and immediate transcription of the patients chart.

12. Which of the following is a unit of measure on a standard prescription?
   a. Millivolts
   b. Micrograms
   c. Millimeters
   d. Amperage

13. Which of the following does not refer to the frequency of administration of patient medication?
   a. qd
   b. bid
   c. po
   d. qid

14. The amount of blood pumped by the heart per minute is called:
   a. Blood pressure
   b. Ejection fraction
   c. Contractility
   d. Cardiac output

15. The Q wave, if present, is always:
   a. Positive
   b. Negative
   c. Isoelectric
   d. Normal

16. The first electrical impulse that is recorded on the ECG paper during a normal cardiac cycle is the:
   a. P wave
   b. T wave
   c. QRS complex
   d. U wave

CHOOSE ONE OF THE FOLLOWING ANSWERS FOR QUESTIONS 17 through 20. MARK THE CORRECT ANSWER ON YOUR ANSWER SHEET.

> A = Wave Form
> B = Interval
> C = Segment
> D = Complex

17. Several wave forms
18. Movement away from the baseline
19. A wave form and a segment
20. A line between wave forms

21. An obese patient was sent to the laboratory for a complete blood count. Of the following veins, which is most likely to be the only one that the can be palpated?
    a. Median cubital vein
    b. Cephalic vein
    c. Basilic vein
    d. Antecubital vein

22. Collection devices used in skin punctures are called:
    a. Capillary tubes
    b. 25 gauge needles
    c. Butterfly sets
    d. Blood culture collection systems

23. How far above the site of draw is the tourniquet placed?
    a. 1-2 inches
    b. 3-4 inches
    c. 4-6 inches
    d. 5-7 inches

24. Which of the following should be used to chill a specimen as it is transported?
    a. Icy water
    b. Frozen blocks of ice
    c. Tepid water
    d. A small freezer unit

25. The tube of choice for glucose testing is:
    a. Light-blue top tube
    b. Red-top tube
    c. Lavender-top tube
    d. Gray-top tube

26. The major parts of a routine urinalysis are:
    a. Physical, Chemical, Microscopic
    b. Chemical, Visual, Culture
    c. Visual, Analytic, Microscopic
    d. Physical, Analytic, Chemical

27. The function of the platelet is to:
   a. Carry nutrients
   b. Cause the blood to clot
   c. Fight infection
   d. Carry oxygen

28. Which reference book is used to check for the correct spelling of drugs:
   a. Standard dictionary
   b. Medical dictionary
   c. Physician's Desk Reference
   d. Current Procedural Terminology

29. Which of the following is the most critical mistake a Phlebotomist can make:
   a. Failing to collect a specimen
   b. Collecting a timed specimen late
   c. A hematoma
   d. Failing to properly identify the patient

30. The EKG records the:
   a. Blood flow through the heart
   b. Heart sounds
   c. Hearts ability to pump
   d. Electrical activity of the heart

Answers to sample test:

1.	A	16.	A
2.	D	17.	D
3.	B	18.	A
4.	B	19.	B
5.	B	20.	C
6.	A	21.	B
7.	C	22.	A
8.	C	23.	B
9.	D	24.	A
10.	B	25.	D
11.	A	26.	A
12.	B	27.	B
13.	C	28.	C
14.	D	29.	D
15.	B	30.	D